9 Silent Assailants Threatening your Heart and How to Beat Them

Paul Boucher

9 Silent Assailants Threatening your Heart and How to Beat Them

This book strives with the new comprehensive approach to cut through the esoteric mystique of medical terms that surround the heart and the arterial system and lets you get your arms around it.

It further provides you with information, so you may be pro-active on your own and loved ones' health care.

This book is not meant to infer that you dismiss your traditional health care professional physician, but hopefully it encourages you to open up a dialogue with him or her.

Paul Boucher

ISBN: 1-4664-8480-2
ISBN-13:   9781466484801

Foreword
By Frederic J. Vagnini, M.D., FACS

When Paul asked me if I would write a foreword for the book he was writing, I immediately, without hesitation, said yes, and furthermore, I would be honored.

I was honored because Paul had been a patient of mine for over two years and is one of the most unique and enjoyable patients I see and someone where the doctor can actually learn from the patient.

I can recall the first time I had a consultation with Paul. As he pulled out his extensive records, I thought this is going to be horrible because I pictured myself staying there for hours reviewing all of these records, which I usually do. However, I was pleasantly surprised with the organization of his extensive medical records, including his past medical history. He had detailed explanations of his diet and exercise program, his drugs and his nutriceuticals. It immediately became an easy task. He was extremely well organized and because of his overwhelming knowledge and research in the area of cardiovascular and metabolic diseases, he always came prepared with lists and charts of his lipid profile, blood chemistries, blood pressure and blood glucose levels.

On Paul's office visits he always gave me a copy of a typed list of questions he wanted to discuss.

On subsequent office visits he had updated his previous reports and he had intelligent questions and diagnostic testing requests. Paul also, through his research, has an excellent understanding of nutrients and drugs. As a matter of fact, recently he reported to me that one of his beta-blockers would be better served by dosing it twice per day rather than once per day and thereby eliminating other drugs, which were affecting his blood glucose.

Overall, after reviewing the book. I highly recommend that the lay person read *9 Silent Assailants*. I think it will help millions of people. Paul has served as an example of one of the mottos, which is, "Your Health is in Your Hands." Accordingly, my recent book, *Countdown Your Age* by McGraw-Hill, 2007 indicated that patients should keep their own records. Paul has followed through with this in excellent fashion and has outstanding medical records.

With regards to his commitments into the management of his own health, it should serve as an example for every individual that an intensive lifestyle, neutriceutical and pharmaceutical program, when necessary, is the way to go.

Frederic J. Vagnini, M.D., FACS

About Dr. Vagnini

Frederic J. Vagnini, M.D., FACS

Dr. Vagnini is a board certified cardiovascular surgeon with over 30 years of surgical experience. His private practice, Heart, Diabetes & Weight Loss Centers of New York, is dedicated to the management of cardiovascular health including blood pressure and cholesterol control, diabetes and obesity. He utilizes natural therapies in conjunction with diet and nutrition, health lifestyle techniques and exercise and nutritional supplementation in treating patients.

Dr. Vagnini is certified by the American Board of Surgery and the American Board of Thoracic Surgery.

Dr. Vagnini is an active, highly respected member of numerous medical societies.

Dr. Vagnini has extensive media experience with hundreds of radio and television appearances. He presently hosts a live call-in show on WOR 710 AM. The show is called "The Heart Show" and airs from 4-5 PM EST Sundays. Dr. Vagnini formerly hosted a national health show on Fox Television.

In the area of print Health Education Dr. Vagnini has written hundreds of articles in the lay literature and has numerous scientific publications. He also publishes a monthly newsletter "Cardiovascular Wellness Newsletter." This publication covers current health news issues with appropriate commentary. The Wellness Newsletter can be ordered through the Center (516 222-2288 or www/vagnini.com).

Books authored and co-authored by Dr. Vagnini:
- *30 Minutes a Day to a Healthy Heart*. Dr. Frederic Vagnini and Silvia Yaeger.
- *Carbohydrate Addict's Healthy Heart Program*. Dr. Richard F. Heller, Dr. Rachael F. Heller, Dr. Frederic Vagnini.
- *The Side Effects Bible*. Dr. Frederic Vagnini and Barry Fox, Ph.D.
- *Overcoming Metabolic Syndrome*. Dr. Frederic Vagnini and Scott Isaacs, M.D.
- *Count Down Your Age*. Dr. Frederic Vagnini and Dave Brunnel.
- *Dr. V's Healthy Heart Plan.*

Heart, Diabetes & Weight Loss Centers of New York
Westbury, NY   Park Avenue, NY
516 222-2288   212 517-2500

Dedication

This book is dedicated to a mother's unconditional love:
to my mother, Jeanette Boucher, and to my beautiful wife
Phyllis and to her mother and my surrogate mother, Shirley
Wolfe.

our raison d'être

our daughters Paulette and Denise Boucher;

our sons: Bruce Solomon, his wife Joan, their children and
our grandchildren Ilana, Daniel and Benjamin;

and Steven Solomon, his wife Jacqueline and their children
and our grandchildren Zachary and Jake.

Acknowledgements

NO MAN IS AN ISLAND

When my wife suggested I stop giving nutritional advice to friends, which had gone on for years over the phone, and write a book, I took her advice.

Since my expertise in writing was limited to tenant/landlord leases, owner/contractor AIA contracts [with riders] and construction specifications, I decided to form three focus groups to send out chapters as I developed them. It is to these unsung heroes [at least in my eyes] that I give my very grateful thanks with putting up with my relentless calls [e.g., is it on track? Should it be left on the tracks? Should I quit my day job?]

Lay person focus group: Toby Hoffman, Bruce Solomon, Jackie Solomon, Steve Solomon, Paulette Boucher, Denise Boucher, Alan Fishman, Ann Forman, Scotty Forman, Arthur Hills, and Professor Dan Levin, C.W Post College.

Medical correctness focus group: Dr. Joan Lebow, Dr. Bill Mesebov, Dr. Robert Ferber, Dr. Clifford Cohen, Dr. Stephen Pruden, and Dr. Frederick Vagnini.

Lab tests focus group: Cattia Lawrence, phlebotomist, Bio Reference Labs.

Book cover design: Paul Boucher and Norman Sonne.

Book cover graphics: Gardenside Graphics, Norman Sonne, Huntington, N.Y.

Editing and proof-reading: Phyllis Boucher (also my best friend). Arthur Hills, Sergeant Major, U.S. Army, retired.

When my research hit a brick wall, I called:

Port Washington Library Research Department, Janet West, Denise Anchico, Jean Bennett, Richard Hausdorff, Kate Monsour, Brooke Salit and Tony Traguardo;

C.W. Post Library and Research Department, Martha Cooney; and

Stony Brook University, Karen Costner.

Last but not least, as this manuscript would not be possible without her, Gisela Zabriskie, typist extraordinaire, All-Round Typing/Translations, 231 Belvedere Drive, Massapequa Park, NY 11762.

With special thanks to Dr. Vagnini [metaphorically speaking], this rocket was poised for lift-off [with partial rocket fuel] until you launched it with your recommendation.

Disclaimer

The author of this book is not a physician and is not dispensing medical advice or prescribing the use of any medical strategy to the reader as a form of treatment for medical problems. On those issues you should seek the advice of your physician. The intent of the author is only to offer information of a general nature for other options so you may be pro-active on your own and loved-ones' health care. In the event you use any of the information from the book for yourself, which is your constitutional right, the author and the publisher assume no responsibility for your actions.

Contents

CHAPTER 1

The Epiphany of My Enlightenments

Whenever I find myself in uncharted waters, which in this case was challenging my doctor's medical advice in my upcoming physical, I reflect on the anxiety of the situation and what circumstances led me here. Somewhere in my self-consciousness I had assigned to my doctor the unconditional acceptance of my mother's advice and nurturing. My doctor became my "Holy Grail" for wellness.

In December of 2000, a cascade of events from my past would combine with my then good friend of 20 years who was also my internist.

> ➤ My interest in health was motivated by my mother's poor health. The poor soul had more than 13 major operations. She had tuberculosis, infantile paralysis [back when the treatment *du jour* was surgery, which left her leg full of scars and a decided limp.], a hysterectomy [probably another unnecessary surgery], pernicious anemia and many other ailments I can't recall. At times I can smell the ether that permeated the hospitals to which I accompanied her.
> My mother passed away in her sleep at 51 years of age, two months after my 25th birthday. The profound loss of my mother motivated me to make a promise to myself not to let that happen to me.
> I soon developed a voracious desire to read Adell Daves's [*an acknowledged authority on vitamin supplements*] books of vitamin supplements and how to lead a healthy lifestyle. Her body of work consists of eight books on the subject.

> - My vitamin reference book was *Earl Mendell's Vitamin Bible*, which soon became my good health bible.

In the summer leading up to my annual pilgrimage to my internist, I serendipitously read a copy of *Heart Sense* whose editor-in-chief was Doctor Stephen Sinatra [as an aside, a cousin of Old Blue Eyes]. As it turns out, he is well recognized in the field of cardiology as well as a certified nutritionist. He was my first introduction to a doctor who practiced alternative medicine.

> *The alternative medicine approach is preventative rather than traditional medicine's approach of treating you after you have the condition. Alternative medicine's preference is nutritional supplements first. In the event they are not effective, they will prescribe prescription drugs in addition to the supplements to be effective synergistically. [The total effect is greater than the sum of the individual effects.]*

Several years later I was fortunate enough to have a consultation with him in his Manchester, Connecticut office.

➤ The following fall I read articles by Doctor Kilmer McCulley of Harvard Medical School, who was later asked to resign because of his work on homocystein and his belief of its importance. [*My sense was that this research had the fingerprints of preventative medicine all over it.*] Dr. McCulley's studies revealed that an amino acid was one of the many culprits of inflammation, which is the breeding ground of plaque formation. He felt homocystein readings over 9 were unacceptable.

➤ Following Dr. McCulley's article I read The Framingham Heart Disease Epidemiology Study which is a landmark study of the factors that contribute to the development of heart disease. Begun in 1948, the study has been following the same group of 5,209 adult volunteers from the city of Framingham, Massachusetts. By keeping track of which people develop heart-related diseases and which do not, vital information to diet and lifestyle was revealed for the first time.

➤ This study is largely responsible for why Americans have become so conscious of the amount of fat in their food and the need for regular exercise. This study is being run by what is now known as the National Heart, Lung and Blood Institute [NHLBI], as well as local universities, physicians and scientists. Before the study, it was widely believed that heart disease was an inevitable result of genetics and aging. Scientists believed it was natural for blood pressure to rise with age as the heart was forced to pump blood through narrowing arteries. The study's findings were among the first to establish a connection between lifestyle choices and a person's heart disease risk level. [Source: http://heart.healthcentersonline.com]

In fact, the term risk factor was coined by Framingham researchers as a direct result of their findings. The Framingham study was instrumental in our modern understanding of how cholesterol levels, smoking, obesity and diabetes contribute to heart disease.

Since heart disease is this country's number two killer with 639,697 deaths [number one are hospital deaths at 783,936], you would expect and depend on the AMA to launch studies on heart attack prevention.

Obviously, at 30,000 dollars a procedure, this is not the case. In 2006 there were 365,000 by-pass operations and approximately 1,000,000 stent procedures. At these prices, the AMA does not need to look too deeply into preventative medicine.

"I will remember that there is art to medicine as well as science and that warmth, sympathy and understanding may outweigh the surgeon's knife or the chemist's drug."

[Abstract of Modern Version of Hippocratic Oath, one of the creeds that they seem to ignore.]

➤ An important medical factor that these studies revealed was that autopsies performed on elderly patients who had died of Alzheimer's disease all had an elevated homocysteine of 13 or higher.

➢ The *Cleveland Clinic Heart Book* section on heart murmurs was very insightful with regard to my former doctor's diagnosis of my heart murmur – "it comes with age." – It should be checked out by an echocardiogram.

The December exam was not the usual *pro forma* exam as it was in past years. At the conclusion of past exams I would dress and go into his consultation room where he told me in his best avuncular manner:

➢ Your x-rays are fine.
➢ Your lab work is fine.
➢ You have the prostate of a 20 year-old.

I expected nothing less. After all, I worked out twice a week, kept my weight down, and ate what I thought at the time was a proper diet, with the occasional fast-food indulgence. I also took, what I thought at the time, was a good regimen of nutritional supplements; drank moderately and got a proper amount of sleep. I will admit, at the mention of my prostate in his consulting room I would shift from side to side in my chair. Frankly, if his passing a Medical Boards depended upon his digital technique on prostates, he would be working at a well known appliance store chain.

This time it would be different:

➢ I had requested a homocystein evaluation included with my regular lab work. *It was 13.5.*

➢ *I had requested he send me to a vascular surgeon,* although my doctor's palpation of my carotid arteries reported them to be fine.
  • Guess what? – *I had a problem with my right internal carotid artery [the one that supplies blood to your brain controlling your left side]. It had a 70% blockage.*

➢ He told me my heart murmur was only a sign of age. His expert medical advice had started to erode. *I didn't buy it; I scheduled an echo cardiogram with a cardiologist. I made a second medical decision – if I don't find another doctor soon, he is either going to kill me or they will name a disease after me.*
  • Another "guess what." *The cardiologist told me, while still on the exam table, I had a problem. He told me I should have my aortic valve replaced because of the plaque build-up, and that there were three types I could select from: bovine, pig, or mechanical. He also suggested a hospital in New York City where they perform minimal invasive procedures [unlike some well-known North Shore hospitals where they cut you open down the center of your sternum, making you a member of the "zipper club"]. He also wanted me to have a stress test ASAP. My ejection factor was 58% { the normal range is 50% to 70%}.*

I later found out the aortic valve problem presented a piggy-back problem.

If you have an aortic valve, or for that matter any heart valve problem, you should take an antibiotic before any dental procedures. *Latest studies suggest this may not be required. I suggest you go over this with your cardiologist.*

If you do not, you could be subjected to the possibility of contracting native valve endocrinitis [NVE]. This is very serious stuff!

I use the antibiotic clindamycin – it doesn't bother my stomach. – I also take a probiotic to restore the intestinal flora the antibiotic destroys. I recommend Metagenics, Ultra Flora Plus DF capsules. Please discuss these issues with your doctor. I will also go into greater depths about pre-biotics in Paul's Cliff Notes.

Driving home from the doctor's exam, I woke up from the nightmare I just came from. My stream of consciousness was racing like the Daytona 500.

- *I now knew why they killed the Greek messenger.*
- *The doctor seemed annoyed that he was interrupted from a conversation with his stock broker to be called in for his expertise in viewing the screen on the torture rack they had me on.*
- *He had "that look." You know, that "look": "I gotcha."*
- *He reminded me of an e-mail I once got. "This message has been automatically generated . . .: when he explained my valve options – reply is not necessary.*
- *Maybe I am lucky with this nightmare – Maybe I just brought my car in to the "pep boys" for a tune-up.*
- *His bedside manner was about as sensitive as the butchers working in the slaughterhouses.*
- *Here is a doctor that thinks "TLC" means "Threaten, Leave them Cowering."*
- *It's not enough they explain your problems in medical-speak, none of which I understand, and after you have the "DAH" look on your face, they don't explain in lay speech.*

Then they plunge the knife in a little further with Gestapo-style psychology [in case you were in too much of a shock to pay attention on the first go-round] by putting the fear of God in you. Those five heart-racing words – You'll die if you don't:
- loose weight or get a gastric by-pass.
- get a stress test today.
- get an angiogram now.
- get a by-pass.
- get this removed.
- don't get this amputated.
- stop smoking.

I am sure the laundry list of threats goes on and on.

In my case, he gave me the bad news while I was lying on the table half dressed with him standing over me and looking down at me. As if I weren't interested enough by that intimidating choreography, he then tells me I need a valve job.

Hey Doc, how about the TLC method!
- *Tell me to get dressed and meet him in his consultation room.*
- Tell me I have a problem with my aortic valve but I am asymptomatic [*no symptoms of a problem*]. We have time especially if your stress test is negative.
- He could then discuss the pros in my case:
  ➢ I am not a smoker.
  ➢ My weight is fairly good.
  ➢ My blood work is excellent.
  ➢ My ejection factor [EF] is 58%, well within the normal range of 50% to 70%. This indicates you have no damage to your left ventricle.
- He then should have explained what that means.

Source: *http://www.chfpatients.com/fag.ef.htm*

What Exactly is EF, Anyway ?

You really have to follow this to understand what's going on with your heart. Come on, it ain't rocket science! Your heart circulates blood through 2 separate systems. The two chambers on top [atriums] are receiving stations for blood. The two lower chambers [ventricles] are pumping stations.

Your left ventricle forces oxygen-rich blood into your arteries, which carries it throughout your body. The blood returns to the right atrium, which passes it down to the right ventricle. The right ventricle pumps this blood to the lungs where it picks up the oxygen. The oxygen-rich blood then returns to the left atrium, which dumps it into the left ventricle, and the cycle repeats. Valves between the chambers prevent "backwash."

When the left ventricle contracts, forcing blood out into the body, it's called "ejection" since it is "ejecting" the blood out into your arteries. Since the big pumper on the lower left is the one that pushes blood throughout your body, that is where they usually measure heart function—the left ventricle.

That's the "ejection" part. The "fraction" part is because that pumping chamber [the left ventricle] never quite manages to pump all the blood inside it—there's always a little bit left behind that lies around waiting for the next contraction. The amount your left ventricle does pump out per beat is called the "ejection fraction." It's X% [the amount pumped out] of the total amount of blood in the ventricle per heart beat.

Gimme a Number

If your heart pumps out 55% or more of the blood in your left ventricle on each beat, you have good heart function. When it falls below 55% on each beat, you're slipping. That means, your heart muscle is too weak to force as much blood out on each contraction as it should.

There is also an ejection fraction for the right ventricle. This measures how well it is pumping blood back to your lungs to pick up oxygen. It is called RVEF and is normally lower than LVEF. Around here, that's what we mean by EF.

Low EF and Mortality

If your EF measured low—say under 35%--this does not mean you are more likely to die! EF is not a predictor of death. So, don't let a low EF panic you! Instead, work on raising it with **meds therapy, low-sodium diet, well-planned exercise**, and other life style changes such as not smoking, not drinking and losing excess weight.

> *I vowed "if," and I said "if," this was not a nightmare and this*
> *came to pass, that's the last time this doctor gets a crack at me!*

Leading up to these events, I was a once-a-year physical exam guy unless something else came up. This meant I had my blood pressure taken once a year. It was always 130/70 and I was told that was fine. As you read on, this was not fine but pre-hypertension, especially someone like me with aortic valve and carotid artery problems.

I passed my stress test, left my traditional doctor, and went to an <u>alternative internist</u> who, unfortunately, relocated within six months.

I had to come up with a strategy to attempt further plaque from developing and perhaps reverse it. At this point I had read every article about the Cleveland Clinic's Dr. Nissen's work in this area. It was exactly what I wanted to do—stop plaque from developing and possibly reverse the plaque. I will discuss in depth his studies and latest findings in the chapter, "Is Traditional Mainstream Medicine Heading for a Crisis?"

I asked my new revolving-door physician to put me on 10mg of Zetia as my cholesterol was ranging from a low of 176 to a high of 227. [This was based on my research on side effects of Zetia as opposed to stronger statins.] I had him also prescribe a diuretic to stabilize my blood pressure and get it in the 120 range.

I was, at this point, concerned with the possibility of a stroke and consulted with five cardiologists [including Dr. Sinatra] before selecting an alternative medicine cardiologist I felt comfortable with.

So here I was, 65 years old feeling like I was at the airport when my ship sailed. I had a tight aortic valve [see, I'm learning Doctor speak] and a carotid artery that was dangerously close to stroking out.

I felt time was not on my side regarding the plaque progression which had gone on too long over many years – *if my former medical "Holy Grail" is within earshot: "thanks."*

In reading more in-depth of Dr. McCulley's hypotheses [*an assumption made in order to test the logical or empirical consequences*] regarding homocysteine creating inflammation in your arterial system which, in turn, was a breeding ground for plaque, all of my readings convinced me of that hypothesis.

Unfortunately, my former doctor never requested a lab report on homocysteine – until that fateful day last year when I requested it. Subsequently it came back at 13.5.

I was now in the Framingham Studies illustrious company [*most lab reports' high range for homocysteine is 15*]. **I had a big-time plaque problem to deal with.** I felt, and still do, that it was caused by the undiscovered high homocysteine I had.

Ruminating over this dilemma in my mind, I still could not accept that this happened – *no, I was not in denial!*

I had kept the information of my cholesterol lab reports for fourteen years of my 20-year hitch with my former doctor.

Cholesterol	222	safe range below	200	over 22
HDL	55	must be above	40*	over 15
Triglycerides	132	must be below	151	under 19
LDL	144	should be below	100	over 44
LDL/HDL Ratio	4.18	should be below	5.0*	under .82

*Value on HDL was lowered to 35, LDL/HDL ratio lowered to 4.2.

Cholesterol years back, under 300 was considered a safe range, now it's below 200; now blood pressure of 130/80 is considered pre-hypertension. Now 120/80 and below is normal.

Due to the electronic ages database medical records-keeping, former medical standards are being adjusted up or down as statistics warrant.

- It's no secret HDL – or high density lipoprotein – helps protect against heart attack, stroke and other forms of cardiovascular disease.
- If you use the former standard of 40, it was 15 points better. If you use the new standard of being above 35, it was 20 points better.
- I have read that if there is an increase of just 10 percent in your HDL, you could lower your cardiovascular risk by 20 to 30%.

For gosh sakes, I was 27.5% better . According to that hypothesis I shouldn't have any plaque. I now fell out of the category of "one size fits all."

If I believed in all of my research about the effectiveness of statins stopping plaque progression – and in some cases reversing it – as substantiated in Cleveland Clinic's famous "reversal study" conducted by Dr. Nissen, I had to pursue a more aggressive statin therapy.

Now that I mapped out that strategy, all I had to do was deal with a hungry surgeon who wanted to replace my aortic valve – this doctor did not do carotid arteries, and had no interest in them or the possibility of an impending stroke. Silly me, I was hoping for a doctor who was interested in the whole me, not just a body part. *Who knew? I strongly felt he needed my fee so his son could complete his last semester at Wharton Business School and receive his MBA. He probably thought he would then get a family discount on his future stock ventures. You've got to hand it to this guy – always thinking!*

I felt time was on my side in the sense that I was asymptomatic and my ejection rate of my heart was high normal. I do not want you to think I was flying blind. I typed a medical bio including medications, vitamins and exercises and attached all my prior tests and sent them to my daughter-in-law, an internist, who was the clinic director for the Cambridge Medical Group in Boston. I wanted her and the staff cardiologist to look things over. Their cardiologist felt I should continue what I was doing and find a cardiologist near me.

➢ *My new cardiologist gave me a second echocardiogram on January 19, 2005, approximately one year later.*
  • *My ejection factor had risen to 68%. I feel this improvement can be credited to riding a recumbent bike eight miles, seven days a week plus my new vitamin regimen and exercise program.*

➢ *My left atrium was not enlarged. That meant to me, based on readings I have done, that although they wanted to replace my aortic valve, it was unnecessary at this time because I was not stressing my heart and I was doing quite well. If I could stop the plaque calcification, I would be headed in the right direction. I felt this was my silver lining.*

Experiencing these tests was not a problem, but their results was like being struck by lightning. Somewhere there was a vague silver lining. I was 65 years old, but felt like 40. I had never been sick a day in my life. Since my mother's illnesses, the birth of my children and the occasional visiting of an ill friend or relative, I have not been in a hospital.

Several weeks after the battery of tests had been performed and the results became known, I was completely disillusioned with my long-term friend and his medical incompetence. I sent him a letter authorizing him to send my medical records to my new internist. He never called to question my actions. That was five years ago. **[Some friend! Some doctor!]**.

That day, after I left his office five years ago, I decided after the bitter disappointment I had experienced with my good friend and doctor, <u>I had to and would become my own health advocate</u>.

In order for the reader to gain confidence and to recognize my credibility in writing this book, the reader has only to realize the journey I had been propelled on since my mother's passing. My original research into this subject, which was further galvanized by my own naiveté and self deception in selecting an internist who has a renowned practice adjacent to the LIJ Hospital in New Hyde Park, New York, was falsely thinking that he must be well qualified.

As it turns out, you can see how wrong that judgment was. The silver lining again! Turning into my own health advocate has led me on a relentless pursuit of researching the following in greater depth:

- ➢ The comprehensive benefit of vitamin supplements and probiotics.
- ➢ The benefits of high fiber foods, although I thought I ate adequate fruits and vegetables.
- ➢ The high and low glycemic food factor and the effect on insulin response.
- ➢ A consistent workout routine with stretching.
- ➢ Researching the histories of:
  1. Herbs
  2. Pharmacopeias
  3. Vitamins, pro biotics
  4. Medicine.

I have read the following periodicals, which I subscribe to, and books which have galvanized my knowledge of healthy living:

Periodicals
- o Doctor Louis J. Ignarro (Nobel Laureate in medicine): *No More Heart Disease*
- o Doctor Thomas E. Levy: *Stop America's #1 Killer*
- o Doctor Stephen Sinatra: *Heart Sense*, later retitled *Heart Health and Nutrition*
- o Doctor Robert Jay Rowers: *Second Opinion*
- o Doctor Julian Whitaker: *Health and Healing*
- o Doctor James Balch: *Prescription of Healthy Living*
- o Tufts University: *Health and Nutrition Letter*
- o Johns Hopkins University: *Medical Letter: Health After 50*
- o Cleveland Clinic: *Heart Advisory* and *Men's Health Advisory*
- o *Harvard Health Letter*
- o *Nutrition Action Letter*
- o *Bottom Line Health*
- o *Consumers in Health*
- o *Life Extension*

Books:
- o Doctor Dean Ornish: *Program for Reversing Heart Disease*
- o Doctor Stephen Sinatra: *Reverse Heart Disease Now*
- o Doctor Andrew Weil: *Spontaneous Healing*
- o Editors of F.C. & A.: *High Blood Pressure Lowered Naturally*
- o Cleveland Clinic: *Heart Book*
- o Johns Hopkins University: *Medical Guide: Health After 50* and *White Paper: Heart Attack Prevention*
- o Mayo Clinic: *Guide to Alzheimer's Disease*
- o Doctor Mark Hyman: *Ultra Prevention* and *Ultra Metabolism*
- o Doctor Mark Hyman and Mark Liponis, M.D.: *Ultra Prevention*
- o Jean Carter: *Food, Your Miracle Medicine*
- o *Bottom Line Book of Total Health and Wellness*

I was fortunate, and I use the word 'fortunate' because the periodicals and books previously mentioned heightened my awareness and introspection that my body was not, as I previously thought, bullet proof and I needed to be more vigilant and proactive than I had ever been in the past and pursue my new 9 spears strategy.

Note: This chapter or any other chapter in this book is not meant to dispense medical advice or strategies for your health care. It is meant to raise your awareness to be pro-active to other health options which should be discussed with your health care professional.

CHAPTER 2

How Did We Get from Medical Antiquity to Here?

Through the centuries, from the earliest archives, medicine had many surrogate fathers. But Hippocrates [359 B.C.] who was influenced by a Greek culture which was a confluence of many earlier civilizations and cultures was recognized by history as its true father. It would take an encyclopedia to list the medical discoveries from its genesis to modern day medicine. I will touch on defining moments I have researched.

Let's share a brief history tutorial 101 on herbs, vitamins, medicines and pharmacopeias. Herbs were the medicine of Antiquity and were used by the following, among others:

- The Pre-Historic Man
- The Egyptians 2900 B.C.
- The Mesopotamians 2600 B.C.
- The Chinese 2000 B.C.
- The Greeks 300 B.C.
- The Romans 100 B.C.
- Throughout Europe in the Middle Ages.

Before recorded time, the early cavemen practiced a form of pharmacopoeia. They learned from instinct. Through their observances of cool water, leaves, dirt and mud, they could make a soothing poultice application. Their methods were crude; much of their learning, as ours is still today, was based on trial and error.

Medicines dispensed by most American pharmacists during the 19th century were derived from plants and other natural substances. The first United States pharmacopoeia [1820] was also derived from plants and other natural substances and was the work of the medical profession's *Book for Drug Standards* which almost did not pass resolution because of the lack of interest by the medical profession.

Doctor Edward R. Squibb, manufacturing pharmacist and physician, protected its extinction.

The sciences of biology and chemistry had not made significant impacts on the theories of disease. <u>Diseases were classified by their symptoms, not their causes</u>. The big health issues of the day were not heart disease, cancer, obesity, or diabetes; they were smallpox, malaria and childhood illnesses.

Eighteenth century apothecaries practiced as doctors. Most learned to diagnose medical conditions and compound medications through an apprenticeship. Surgeons also learned their trade through an apprenticeship.

It would take several volumes to describe medical discoveries from its genesis to modern day medicine. I will not even try but I will chronicle the discoveries of the more and not so familiar defining moments.

- 1601. One of the most interesting bits of information I researched was the *first unintentional controlled study*—performed in 1601 by Captain James Lancaster. He captained one ship among a fleet that set sail in April, and by the time they had arrived at their destination in September of that same year, the other ships had been so devastated by scurvy that Lancaster's men, healthy and whole, had to assist the other ships, explaining he had brought on board bottles of lemon juice and every man took three spoonfuls each morning—this giving way to British sailors' nickname of "limey."
  - *I feel I cannot mention Vitamin C without a word about Doctor Linus Pauling, two-time Nobel Prize winner. Although he never discovered Vitamin C, he was the most vociferous advocate Vitamin C ever had. His body of work included DNA immunology, sickle cell anemia, genetics, evolution and human health.*
- 1636. Harvard University was founded.
- 1705. Giovanni Morgagni an assistant professor of anatomy in Bologna, Italy had collected several hundred anatomy studies and *had inadvertently performed the second unintentional controlled study.*
- *These are the only two unintentional controlled studies in my research which in essence are anecdotal, which I will discuss in a subsequent chapter.*

<u>Note</u>: Major medical accomplishments worth mentioning are listed in the Appendix so as not to bore readers not interested in these facts.

Pharmacopoeia

While compounding and selling drugs is as old as civilization, its background in the United States developed along these time lines.

- 1810. Patent medicines were one of the largest industries in the U.S.
- 1820. The first United States Pharmacopoeia [U.S.P.] was the work of the medical profession. It was the first book of drug standards from a professional source to have achieved a nation's acceptance.
- During the Civil War the Union army required large quantities of quality opium, quinine and Ergot. This established companies like Eli Lilly and E. R. Squibb. During this era, Park Davis and Up-John were also emerging pharmaceutical companies. Their scientific staffs concentrated on standardized preparations and rarely did research. Source: College Pharmacy
- *In 1993, Squibb reported 11.1 billion in revenues.*
  Source: *Shaping the Industrial Century*, Chandler.
- In 1887, the "U.S.P." was in danger of dissolution due to the lack of interest of the medical profession. The advocacy by Dr. Edward R. Squibb, a manufacturing pharmacist as well as a physician, took the problem to "the American Pharmaceutical

Association" convention which formed a "Committee of Revision." The "U.S.P." then surged to a new importance.

- 1903. Until 1903 the drug industry was based on a few well known active ingredients.
- 1905. The Pure Food & Drug Act prohibiting the manufacture and distribution of adulterated drugs.
- 1938. The FDA Act, when support data mainly determined by drug firms themselves were submitted to the FDS for approval, the FDA had to respond within 60 to 180 days. If not, the data was automatically approved.
- 1940. Controlled studies were established in the mid- to late-forties and became "the gold standard" for judging the validity of all prescription drugs.
  - *This kind of study supposedly eliminated subjective conclusions based on the interpretation of the doctor or the patient. [Author] In my opinion, I believe this was the beginning of a 180 degree turning point by the medical profession. They used a nihilistic approach and abandoned the bed stone of an earlier pharmacology, an anecdotal experience with vitamins and nutritional supplements proven through trial and error through the millenniums, for the more profitable prescription drugs. They felt they were more expedient, completely ignoring the disastrous side effects new therapy might bring that had not endured the test of time. [Nihilism: a view posed that traditional values and beliefs are unfounded and that existence is senseless and useless.]*
  - *I believe that this was the first footnote of the future influence of the stranglehold that the pharmaceutical industry would get on the medical profession.*
  - *It's also my opinion this was the genesis that "before the fact" [prevention] treatment of medical conditions were pushed to the background. It was easier to stop the bleeding after it started than before it started.*
  - *It's my further opinion it was in the pharmaceutical industry's [Big Pharmas] best interest to pursue profit making drugs (which could be patented), not natural substances which could not.*
- 1950. By the end of the 1950's the pharmaceutical company had changed beyond recognition as it developed antibiotics, steroids, antihistamines and tranquilizers in addition to new drugs for the heart, lung disease, ulcers, cancers, diabetes, pain control and other ills which were also followed by new vaccines.

The face of medicine had also changed.

This period contributed to strict regulations for clinical drug testing. Under the new law, pharmaceutical companies were required to get FDA approval prior to any tests of new drugs on human subjects. Approval was also required to distribute new drugs to other states for clinical research, which was only given after comprehensive results of animal tests were furnished. Before pharmaceutical companies were permitted to put a new drug onto the market, they had to prove its efficacy and that manufacturers' claims for it were accurate. Information about side effects, contraindications, and effectiveness of the drug had to be included in advertising materials. The FDA had six months to review applications as well as the right to extend its review period indefinitely.

- *1962. The over-the-counter "OTC" sleeping pill Thalidomide caused 8,000 deformed babies worldwide.*
- *1969. The FDA reported that half of about 500 over-the-counter [OTC] product samples they examined were not effective.*
- *1985 spurred the complaints of unfair FDA handling of drug applications; the House of Representatives began investigating FDA practices and the generic drug industry as a whole. <u>A plethora of corrupt activities was discovered, including payoffs, disregard of agency guidelines, even rigged pre-approval tests of drugs. FDA officials served prison terms after being found guilty of accepting bribes and the half-dozen generic companies found guilty of fraud and deceptive practices were closed.</u> The FDA generic division was reorganized from the ground up and onsite, pre-approval inspections of drug companies were begun.*
  Source: *D&B Gale Industry Handbook.*
- *2004. Merck & Co. withdrew its Vioxx pain drug from the market after class action law suits, and their study showed the drug posed high cardiac stroke risks.*

1/24/07 – RETURN OF THE DRUG COMPANY PAYOFFS

Two excessively lenient court decisions have allowed the manufacturers of brand-name drugs to resume the underhanded practice of paying generic competitors to keep their drugs off the market. It is a costly legal loophole that needs to be plugged by Congressional legislation.

The problem arises when a generic manufacturer tries to take its drug to market before the patent on a brand-name drug has expired by arguing that its product does not infringe upon the patent or that the patent is invalid. Huge sums of money are at stake, especially with the blockbuster drugs whose annual sales can exceed a billion dollars.

Rather than risk it all, a brand-name manufacturer may choose to pay its generic competitor substantial compensation to drop its challenge and delay marketing its drug. Both companies make out handsomely. The big losers are consumers and the public and private insurers that must continue to pay monopoly prices for the brand-name drugs.

The Federal Trade Commission, which has been waging a valiant fight, succeeded for several years in eliminating such settlements. But two appeals court decisions in 2005 held that they are a legitimate way to resolve patent disputes. And sure enough, the F.T.C. reported later that year—after a five-year hiatus—brand-name companies made three such do-not-compete settlements in the fiscal year 2005 and fourteen more last year.

The pharmaceutical industry contends that the settlements are a reasonable way to resolve disputes and that they often result in bringing generic drugs to market before a patent has expired, albeit not as soon as the generic company wanted. The industry argues that regulators and the courts should judge such settlements on a case-by-case basis.

Our own hunch is that the better approach for Congress to take as it moves toward corrective legislation would be a "bright line" prohibition against making any payments to delay introduction of a generic drug. That would set a clear standard and enhance the likelihood that consumers would get a chance to benefit from real competition in the pharmaceutical market.

Source: *The New York Times*, 1/24/07

2.2.07 – STUDIES OVERDUE FOR DRUGS IN USE

Drugmakers have yet to begin more than two out of every three pending studies that they promised to do after their products were approved by U.S. regulators.

The Food and Drug Administration determined that 899 or 71 percent of 1,259 post-approval studies hadn't been started as of Sept. 30, according to date posted recently on the agency's web site. The numbers do not include completed studies.

To receive FDA approval, drugmakers often agree to perform additional studies of safety dosing and other matters after medications come to market. The studies are usually voluntary, and the FDA can't impose fines for failing to conduct them. Some consumer groups and lawmakers are pushing for legislation to give the FDA more authority over the studies.

"How can the FDA claim it is committed to improving the drug safety when it can't even get drugmakers to do the studies they promise?" said Bill Vaughan, senior policy analyst with Consumers Union in Washington, D.C. in a statement. "Should consumers really feel safe when two out of three studies aren't being done and the FDA doesn't even have the authority to get them done?"

Members of Congress have criticized the FDA's oversight of drug safety in recent years. As studies linked antidepressants to suicide risk for children and painkillers to elevated chances of heart attacks, doctors say post-approval studies may be needed to fully assess the risks because some dangers don't emerge until products are widely used.

"The FDA is seeking ways to work with drugmakers to carry out the studies," agency spokeswoman Susan Cruzan said in an e-mail response to questions. "The agency also is trying to improve its ability to track and monitor the studies," she said.

"Drugmakers are committed to completing the studies," said Alan Goldhammer, Deputy Vice President for Regulatory Affairs at the Pharmaceutical Research and Manufacturers of America, an industry group in Washington. "Sometimes companies have difficulty finding enough patients to participate," he said.

Source: *Bloomberg News*, 2/2/07.

- *1990's. By the mid-90's Pfizer's net income alone surpassed 1.3 billion.*
- *2005. Drug sales worldwide reached 605 billion.*

Source: *Market Share,* reporter Robert S. Lazich.

The negative news media articles bashing nutritional supplements are for the most part based on flawed studies.

The release of these articles is ultimately sponsored by the Big Pharma puppetmaster while the AMA turns its back.

For example, one such study surrounding the storm of controversy about vitamin E is a study by Johns Hopkins, a recipient of Big Pharma yearly grants:

> *The Johns Hopkins team looked at 19 studies carried out between 1993 and 2004 involving more than 136,000 people. People who took daily vitamin E doses exceeding 400 "International units" (IU) per day (equivalent to about 270 mg) had an increased risk of death by about 10% compared with those who did not.*

> *Dr. Robert Verkerk, executive director of the Alliance for Natural Health, said: "Negative publicity about vitamin E, which is likely to follow as a result of misinterpretations over the science behind the Johns Hopkins study, could scare people unnecessarily and stop them using important food supplements."*

> *Dr. Richard Slow, a lecturer in the cardiovascular division at King's College London, said: "The medical community and the public should treat these findings with a degree of caution since this analysis combines the results from a very broad spectrum of epidemiological studies carried out over 38 years, utilizing doses of vitamin E supplementation between 16.5 to 2000 IU per day."*
> Source: BBC News.

> *I believe the reverse effect also pertains to some of the conflicting data we see on Vitamin E. We all know that cardiovascular disease (CVD) is the leading cause of death in the industrialized world. And vitamin E studies have shown that a high dietary intake of vitamin E can result in a lower incidence of cardiovascular disease – including cardiovascular death. But placebo-controlled clinical trials with supplemental vitamin E showed little or no benefit.*
> Source: BBC News.

> ***In all the major trials on vitamin E, pure alpha-tocopherol was used as a supplement.*** *My theory has been that pure supplemental alpha-tocopherol, which lacks the gamma-tocopherol that accompanies dietary vitamin E foods, could have an adverse health effect. The problem is, if you take high-dose alpha-tocopherol and aren't getting enough gamma-tocopherol in your diet or in supplement form, you risk a pro-oxidant effect from vitamin E. Another problem is that taking large doses of alpha-tocopherol can deplete the gamma-tocopherol in your system, so taking alpha-tocopherol alone can hurt rather than help – just when you thought you were doing the right thing.*

You see, only gamma-tocopherol has the potent antioxidant activity to eradicate the dangerous peroxynitrite radical that can damage cell membranes and accelerate the aging process. Too much alpha-tocopherol wipes out gamma receptors. But it doesn't take much of a dose of gamma-tocopherol to offset any negative effect of alpha-tocopherol.

<u>Clinical researchers demonstrated that, in patients with cardiovascular disease, plasma levels of gamma-tocopherol are low. In one study lasting seven years and including 34,686 postmenopausal women, the researchers showed that diets rich in gamma-tocopherol sources were inversely correlated to death from cardiovascular disease.</u> In other words, postmenopausal women eating more nuts, almonds and wheat germ had less cardiovascular death than women taking supplemental alpha-tocopherol. So, even a small amount of dietary gamma-tocopherol can make a huge difference in reducing cardiac risk.

If you're investing your time and money to take vitamin E, you don't want a reverse effect. So, if you're one of the millions of people taking high-dose alpha-tocopherol supplements (greater than 400 units daily), then be sure to complement that supplement with natural sources of gamma-tocopherol found in wheat germ, palm oil, sesame seeds, almonds, pecans, peanuts and Brazil nuts.

An even better approach to guarantee that you get the right balance of tocopherols is to take them in a supplement that contains mixed tocopherols. <u>I endorse vitamin E preparations containing a total of 200-400 units of mixed tocopherols including vital gamma-tocopherol (the amount and proportion of gamma to alpha tocopherol is not important as far as we know).</u> It's also extremely important to take natural vitamin E, and not the synthetic type. <u>Synthetic vitamin E labels are clearly marked with a "DL," (which in my mind stands for "darn lousy," so it's very easy to tell the difference.</u>
Source: Dr. Stephen Sinatra, *Heart, Health and Nutrition.*

Everyone is brainwashed [by the venerable American Medical Association and the Pharmaceutical Industry's (the Machiavellian puppeteer with a stranglehold on the AMA) richly funded advertising programs on a daily basis].

Don't let your health be lost to statistics and advertising.

<u>Attention readers</u>: I felt you would appreciate [as general background] reading the following chapters before reading "Nine Silent Assailants" as sort of an ABCs primer. If not, skip to the chase.

Note: This chapter or any other chapter in this book is not meant to dispense medical advice or strategies for your health care. It is meant to raise your awareness to be pro-active to other health options which should be discussed with your health care professional.

CHAPTER 3

Is Traditional Mainstream Medicine Heading for a Crisis?

Integrated/alternative medicine is becoming a recognized movement and growing rapidly being mainly fueled by the baby boomer generation.

According to the book *Death by* Medicine, by Gary Null, Ph.D.; Carolyn Dean, M.D.; Martin Feldman, M.D.; Debora Rasiom, M.D.; and Dorothy Smith, Ph.D., U.S. hospitals had 783,936 deaths due to iatrogenic deaths: *induced inadvertently by a physician or surgeon or by medical treatment or diagnostic procedures.* Of that figure a recent study concluded that doctors cause 305,000 hospital deaths each year due to adverse drug reactions –the third leading cause of death in the United States after heart disease and cancer [heart disease 699,697, cancer 553,281].

ANNUAL PHYSICAL AND ECONOMIC COST OF MEDICAL INTERVENTION

Condition	Deaths	Cost	Author
Hospital ADR [adverse drug reaction]	106,000	$ 12 billion	Lazarou Suh
Medical Error	98,000	$ 2 billion	IOM
Bedsores	115,000	$ 55 billion	Xakellis Barczak
Infection	88,000	$ 5 billion	Weinstein MMWR
Malnutrition	108,800	---------------	Nurses Coalition
Outpatient ADR [adverse drug reaction]	199,000	$ 77 billion	Starfield Weingart
Unnecessary Procedures	37,136	$ 122 billion	HCUP
Surgery-Related	32,000	$ 9 billion	AHRQ
TOTAL	**783,936**	**$282 billion**	

Source [abstracted]: http://www.wnho.net/deathbymedicine.htm

That's 45,063 less deaths than all the soldiers killed in the Civil War [510,700], World War I [116,708], Korean War [54,246] and the Vietnam War [58,219].

The total of these wars was 17 years, as opposed to the total hospital deaths of 783,936 during one year.

That also equates approx. six fully loaded A380 Air Buses fully loaded crashing every other day for a year.

Of the 783,936 hospital deaths, 304 were caused by adverse drug reaction.

The National Safety Board statistics for accidental highway deaths for 2006 were 108,694.

This translates into the sobering statistics that you have a 70% less chance of dying, being a national highway statistic, than being in a U.S. hospital and dying from an adverse drug reaction.

Those statistics are pretty scary. You certainly don't get adverse drug reactions from vitamins and nutritional supplements and staying out of hospitals.

Approximately 150 million people use supplements each year, but just 240 deaths have been attributed to supplements from 1994 to 2004 [the most recent years for which we have statistics]. That averages out to about 22 supplement-related deaths each year. What's more, most of those deaths were linked to products that contained ephedra (*which was subsequently banned by the FDA – a principal acting amphetamine-like compound can powerfully stimulate the nervous system and heart*). And the problem wasn't actually the ephedra itself—it was the use of ephedra products in combination with caffeine, a practice that the product's label warned against. The result was a risky recipe that could, and did, cause deadly ventricular fibrillation
Source: *Heart, Health & Nutrition*, March 2007.

ANNUAL UNNECESSARY MEDICAL EVENTS STATISTICS

Unnecessary Events	People Affected	Iatrogenic Events
Hospitalization	8.9 million	1.78 million
Procedures	7.5 million	1.3 million
TOTAL	**16.4 million**	**3.08 million**

The enumerating of unnecessary medical events is very important in our analysis. Any medical procedure that is invasive and not necessary must be considered as part of the larger iatrogenic picture. Unfortunately, cause and effect go unmonitored. The figures on unnecessary events represent people ["patients"] who are thrust into a dangerous healthcare system. They are helpless victims. Each one of these 16.4 million lives is being affected in a way that could have a fatal consequence. Simply entering a hospital could have the following:

1. Of 16.4 million people, 2.1% chance of a serious adverse drug reaction (186,000).
2. Of 16.4 million people, 5-6% chance of acquiring a nosocomial infection (489,500).
3. Of 16.4 million people, 4-36% chance of having an iatrogenic injury in hospital [medical error and adverse drug reactions] (1.78 million).
4. Of 16.4 million people, 17% chance of procedure error (1.3 million).

All the statistics above represent a one-year time span. Imagine the number over a ten-year period.
Source [abstracted]: http://www.wnho.net/deathbymedicine.htm.

Hospitals should be viewed the same as parachutes: you definitely need them, but pray you never use them.

Aug. 2004   *Newsday Health*
72 deaths during a three-year period caused by statin drugs; 20 were linked to Baycol. The FDA withdrew it from the market the same year.

Nov. 2004   *Newsday Health* – Washington Bureau
             98,000 Americans die each year from preventable medical errors.

Sept. 2005   *Newsday Health*
             "Beta Blockers"
             Researchers followed 735 patients over three years; 20% of the group with two genetic variations died using Beta blockers compared to those without them. The gene variations made the drug less effective and may affect more than half the 1.7 million Americans who are hospitalized each year with mild heart attacks.

2005   *USA Today*
Mar. 2006   A popular antibiotic (Tequin). About 5,000 prescriptions are written a day and are at risk for blood sugar problems.

Apr. 2006   *Newsday Health*
             Celebrex taken basically to relieve pain raises risk of colon cancer and raises risk of heart problems.

             Washington Post
             At least 1.5 million Americans are sickened, injured and killed each year by avoidable errors in prescribing, dispensing and taking medications, the Institute of Medicine concludes in their report.

Another study recently suggested something as simple as taking a daily multivitamin to protect against disease of aging could save Medicare $1.6 billion over 5 years.

The doctors simply miss the prevention opportunities to suggest vitamins to their patients during office visits, e.g.:

- *They don't study vitamins and nutritional supplements in medical school.*
- *The huge financial resources of the pharmaceutical companies' representatives making weekly calls with free samples and offers of free trips and other perks mentioned by Dr. Jerome D. Kassierer in his statement to the Ways and Means Committee.*
- *The doctors' reluctance to consider two approaches – prescription drugs and vitamins are better than drugs alone.*
- *The next statement by Jerome P. Kassierer, M.D. to the House Committee must have tempted "Big Pharma" to put a bounty on his head.*

HOUSE COMMITTEE ON WAYS AND MEANS

Statement of Jerome P. Kassirer, M.D., Professor, Tufts University School of Medicine, Boston, Massachusetts.

Testimony Before the Subcommittee on Health of the House Committee on Ways and Means, July 21, 2005:

I am Jerome P. Kassirer, M.D., Distinguished Professor at Tufts University School of Medicine in Boston; Adjunct Professor of Medicine and Bioethics at Case Western Reserve University School of Medicine in Cleveland; former Editor-in-Chief of the *New England Journal of Medicine*, and sole author of the book, *On the Take: How Medicine's Complicity with Big Business Can Endanger Your Health.*

Extracts from Dr. Kassirer's testimony:

➤ Over 80% of the more than $20 billion yearly of advertising expenses of the pharmaceutical industry is directed at doctors and other health care professionals. There is nothing fundamentally wrong with advertising products, but when financial incentives yield inappropriate or dangerous care, when they inordinately raise the cost of care, and when their effect is to damage the trust of patients in the profession, they have gone too far. **You could never get this teacher-to-student ratio in the most expensive private school in the world.**
   - *To make sure they covered all of their bases, the pharmaceutical industry spends another $200 million on 625 lobbyists which is the largest lobby with the largest budget in Washington, D.C. to woo the 100 members of our Congress and the 435 members of our House of Representatives.*
   Source: http://www.AARP.org/bulletin/medicare/articles/on2003-06-23-drugindustry.html?print-yes.

➤ An FDA panel of 10 members who had financial arrangements with the industry voted 9 to 1 to return Vioxx back to the market despite its being recognized for cardiovascular toxicity.

➤ FDA approval of Natrecor for patients with acute episode of heart failure reached an estimated annual sales of almost $700 million. It is a widely given drug by infusion routinely and repeatedly in doctors' offices. Each visit is $500 to $600. According to expert cardiologists there is no data that routine use is beneficial.

➤ There is increasing evidence that Natrecor (*an intravenous medication*) damages the kidneys and may even increase the death rate.

➤ Heart failure is a common condition and infusing one patient a day could yield $150,000 a year to a physician's bottom line.
   - *Speaking of physicians' greed, a golfing buddy of mine by the name of John Orlick (he was one of the arresting officers on the narcotic squad of*

the famous Popeye Doyle in the French Connection in 1971) said his former cardiologist recommended the need of a pacemaker for John.

- *He got a second opinion and after numerous tests he was told by his new cardiologist that he did not need one. By the way, the cost of a pacemaker is approximately $5,500 or more, depending on who is doing the procedure.*

➤ At the present, the pharmaceutical industry pays for well over half the expenses of doctors' continuing education. Medical centers, as well as medical schools, rely on drug company funding.

➤ Drug companies also pay individual doctors to speak at national meetings, medical center conferences and at restaurant back rooms.

➤ Although the speakers are usually told that they are not obligated to mention the sponsor's drugs, there is a natural sense of obligation to reciprocate for the $750 to $4,000 honorarium.

➤ In 2004, the *Wall Street Journal* reported a number of pharmaceutical company-sponsored meetings and talks that featured doctors as speakers had grown to nearly 240,000.

➤ Even more worrisome than the effect of bias on the part of individual speakers is the potential effect of financial conflict of interest on the development of clinical practice guidelines, the professional society's advice to practicing doctors about the treatment of certain conditions. Similar to the broad influence of FDA decisions on drug use, a statement from the American College of Physicians or the American Neurological Association on the treatment of migraine, for example, would have a major impact on the use of the drugs recommended in a guideline report. Both the public and profession paid close attention one year ago when a clinical practice guideline issued by three prestigious organizations, the American Heart Association, the American College of Cardiology, and the National Institutes of Health, unveiled guidelines for cholesterol.

➤ The levels were so stringent that millions of Americans at risk of heart disease would have to take costly statin drugs to meet the proposed low limits. What the three organizations didn't reveal was that most panel members who helped write the recommendations had financial ties to the pharmaceutical companies that stood to gain enormously from increased use of statins. The extent of the connections was stunning: of the nine members of the panel that wrote the guidelines, six had each received research grants, speaking honoraria or consulting fees from at least three and in some cases all five of the manufacturers of statins; only one had no financial links. In response to criticism of the panel composition, the Heart Association said that the policy had been reviewed by many others, not just formulated by nine people, yet they did not disclose the conflicts of any other reviewers. Even if they had, such disclosures would have.

➢ This brief description covers only a small fraction of the consequences of medical-pharmaceutical financial connections.

➢ Flaws in research study design, bias reporting of research and risks to patients in clinical trials constitute other serious consequences.
   • *Let me lead you through a good news/bad news outcome [except for the obvious side effects of statins] and a bad outcome of research design studies and clinical trials.*

High Intensity Statin Therapy May Reverse Atherosclerosis [hardening of the arteries] in coronary disease patients, suggested a study published in the *Journal of the American Medical Association.* Cleveland Clinic researcher Steven E. Nissen, M.D. and colleagues studied 507 patients with mean baseline LDL ("bad") cholesterol level of 143 mg/dl. The patients underwent an initial intravascular ultrasound [IVUSA] to measure their progression of atherosclerosis and received 40 mg daily doses of the cholesterol-lowering drug rosuvastatin [Crestor]. After 24 months, 349 of the study participants underwent a follow-up IVUS. The patients' mean LDL levels decreased by 53.2 percent to 60.8 mg/dl [less than the current recommended target reduction level of 70 mg/dl], while HDL levels rose 14.7 percent to 49 mg/dl according to the study. The improvements in cholesterol levels resulted in significant regression of atherosclerosis, based on the follow-up IVUS results.

Source: *Cleveland Clinic's Men's Health,* 5/2006.

   • We've only decreased , roughly, thirty percent of heart attacks for people on statins. Can we reduce it even further? Our goal would be to decrease it 95 percent, and that is one reason to pursue HDL therapy.
   • The story of a patented HDL began more than two decades ago, when Italian investigators reported that about 40 inhabitants of Limone Sul Garde, a town in Northern Italy, has extraordinarily low HDL levels, so low they were off the scale. Doctors expected that they would have high rates of heart disease, but, instead, it was reported they actually seem to be protected from heart diseases and to live unusually long lives. They called it Apoliprotein or APOA-1.
   • One of the first to study apo-a-1 Milano was Dr. Prediman K. Shah, who directs the atherosclerosis research center at Cedars Sinai Medical Center. He reported it prevented plaque growth in arteries of rabbits and in mice. At higher doses, it even reversed the accumulation of plaque in mice. It took just six weeks.
   • "There was still skepticism at this point," Dr. Shah said. "But we were convinced."
   • There was, however, one patented HDL and Dr. Roger Newton, the president and chief executive of Esperion Therapeutics of Ann Arbor, MI licensed the rights to develop it. Dr. Newton had developed a cholesterol-lowering drug; He was a discoverer of Lipitor, the most prescribed statin

in the United States. His goal in forming Esperion in 1998 was to develop HDL.

- But in the meantime, Pharmacia, now owned by Pfizer, had obtained the patent rights to the HDL they make, known as apoa-1 Milano. Esperion licensed the rights from Pharmacia, and the research began.

- After conducting early tests of the HDL in humans, looking for safety, Esperion approached Dr. Nissen. He had developed a technique, intravascular ultrasound that involves threading a tiny ultrasound camera into arteries and directly observing plaques and precisely measuring their size. Would he direct a small study using that method to use for the drug's effects on plaque?

- Dr. Nissen was dubious. Most studies he participates in go on for two or three years and involve 500 or more subjects to see an effect. This was to last just five weeks and involve about 50 people.

- When he saw the data, he was stunned. "The plaque regressed. A lot. More than has been seen with any drug. He almost fell off his seat. This is just so bizarre and unusual."

- "Until now, the paradigm has been to prevent disease by lowering bad cholesterol," Dr. Nissen said, referring to LDL lowering. "If you get the bad cholesterol low enough, the plaques don't build up in the artery walls. This says you can also remove the disease in the wall of the artery."

- Prior to Pfizer launching a study involving 15,000 patients, Esperion Therapeutics' share rose 35% after announcing the findings of the small study.

Source: *The New York Times*, 11/5/2003. Abstract of story.

- Heart disease is the nation's leading cause of death. The number of Americans suffering heart attacks and strokes has been dropping, in part because of the development of cholesterol-lowering drugs known as statins, which have become one of the most widely used and effective tools in medicine. Those drugs work by lowering levels of low-density lipoprotein or LDL, which is known as the "bad" cholesterol because it accumulates inside arteries. But many patients remain at risk even when their LDL has been brought to a level considered safe.

- Although a number of compounds designed to boost HDL levels are being studied, Torcetrapib was by far the furthest along in development. After initial studies showed the drug was highly effective at raising HDL levels, Pfizer launched a study involving more than 15,000 patients at high risk for heart attack and stroke. Half took torcetrapib along with the statin Lipitor; the other half took Lipitor alone.

Source: *The Washington Post*, 1/28/07. Abstract of Abstracts.

The Bad News

- Manhattan-based Pfizer had expected to sell torcetrapib in combination with Lipitor, which lowered LDL, or bad cholesterol, and is the company's—and the world's—best selling drug. According to Pfizer spokesman Paul Fizhenry, 82 patients taking the combination of torcetrapib died, compared to 51 deaths in the arm of the study where patients were taking Lipitor alone. Each arm of the study had 7,500 patients. Pfizer said that the study didn't raise any questions about Lipitor's safety.

- The world's largest drugmaker said it was told that an independent board monitoring a study for <u>torcetrapib</u>, a drug that raises levels of HDL commonly known as good cholesterol, recommended the termination of the drug's use because of "an imbalance of mortality and cardiovascular events." Pfizer said it is asking all clinical investigators conducting trial to warn patients to stop taking the drug immediately.

    Source: *Newsday*, 1/28/07. Abstract of Abstracts.

➢ "Given the extensive involvement, extracting medicine from the pharmaceutical industry magnet will be extremely difficult, but I believe it must be done." – Dr. Jerome P. Kassirer

    Source: Abstract from http://waysandmeans.house.gov/hearing.
    ASP?formmode=printfriendly&16=2033

Author: Don't forget, that man is a Head Doctor yet!

Note: This chapter or any other chapter in this book is not meant to dispense medical advice or strategies for your health care. It is meant to raise your awareness to be pro-active to other health options which should be discussed with your health care professional.

CHAPTER 4

Experimentation by any other Name is Still Experimentation

Webster's Dictionary says: "the act, process, or practice of making experiments."

There are many levels of experimentation. I will only be discussing three: Dr. Frankenstein's clinical trials, and Paul's trials.

You are mistaken if you think Dr. Frankenstein is only in the movies.
- Most believed that following World War II human experimentation would be viewed as so abhorrent that no one would dare try it again. But as we've seen, human radiation as well as chemical, biological and mind control experiments flourished throughout the 1940s, 1950s and 1960s with little regard for human life. And while much of the research was military, organized medicine was enthusiastically getting into the act itself.
- By 1940, physicians were eager to expand medical databases—and boost their careers in the process—even if it meant performing risky human experiments on everyone from babies to the elderly.

Conventional medical procedure was simply to induce illness in healthy medical research subjects. In studies done from 1951 to 1952, insulin was withheld from diabetic patients for as long as two days so as to induce diabetes. Some became comatose.
- Children were also used widely in medical experiments.
- In 1949 the *Lancet* reported an experiment in which eighty children as young as ten years were fed agenized flour for six months to investigate the toxic effects of agene, an ingredient used in the production of flour.
- A 1953 article in *Clinical* Science details an experiment in which forty-one children aged ten to fourteen, had their abdomens deliberately blistered with cantharide to study the severity of the response to the irritant. In his own words, the author of the study describes the procedure as if he were describing an experiment with lab rats.
- Archives of Pediatrics describe how physicians transmitted Vincent's angina.
- The *Journal of Clinical Investigation* published a report on what today would be considered torture. In 1957, doctors at Children's Hospital in Philadelphia wanted to investigate how blood flows through children's brains. Healthy children, aged three to eleven, were selected for the experiments. The researchers, who note in their article that some of the children had to be restrained by bandaging them to a board, inserted one needle into the femoral artery of the thigh and one into the jugular vein of the neck, which brings blood down from the brain. While the children had the needles secured in their bodies, they were forced to inhale a special gas through a facemask.
- In 1963, a study published in *Pediatrics* stated 113 newborn infants, aged one hour to three days, were used to measure changes in blood pressure and blood flow. The procedure was something one would expect at Dachau concentration camp, not at the University of California's Department of Pediatrics. The doctors would insert, without medication, a catheter via the umbilical artery into the infant's aorta. The infant's feet would then be immersed in ice water and the aortic pressure recorded. Another fifty

infants were strapped to a circumcision board and tilted over the edge of a table so that blood would rush to their heads before blood flow and pressure were measured.

- The *British Medical Journal* about early medical experiments: "Children from orphanages and foundlings were commonly used as subjects for these investigations."
- Literally, every major research hospital was using children for experiments, with little or no indication of parental consent.

1956-1972:   Dr. Saul Krugman of New York University, in a study funded by the Armed Forces Epidemiological Board, injects hepatitis serum into mentally disabled children at Willowbrook School on Staten Island. Krugman has the parents sign an informed consent document which suggests the children will be receiving a vaccine to prevent hepatitis. In 1972, Krugman became President of the American Pediatric Society.

1983:   FDA Common Rule amended to add Special protections for children.
- As recently as 2001, the U.S. Food and Drug Administration [FDA] admitted that its policy to include healthy children in human experiments may have had some unexpected consequences.
- Prisoners were—and still are—used as a steady source of human tests.
- Penitentiaries in Georgia, Oklahoma, Kansas, Mississippi, Ohio, and Pennsylvania became breeding grounds for human subjects who volunteered for experiments in exchange for rewards as small as a pack of cigarettes or, in some cases, a few days shaved from their sentences. Research projects included organ transplantation, medical techniques, injection of liver cancer cells or blood from patients with leukemia, effects of chemicals and drugs on the human body, and exposure to radiation. The March 1964 issue of *Medical News* reported that at Holmesburg Prison in Pennsylvania, nine of ten prisoners were medical research subjects and that throughout the United States the number was in the thousands.

1962-1980:   Pharmaceutical companies conduct phase one safety testing of drugs almost exclusively on prisoners for small cash payments.

1980:   The FDA promulgates 21 CFR 50.44 prohibiting use of prisoners as subjects in clinical trials shifting phase one testing by pharmaceutical companies to nonprison population.
- As if their reputations weren't sullied enough, cancer researchers took another hit when Dr. Linus Pauling, winner of the Nobel Prize in Chemistry and the Nobel Peace Prize said:
    "The way in which the American people have been betrayed by the cancer establishment, the medical profession, and the government are shocking. Everyone should know that the war on cancer is largely a fraud and a sham, and that the National Cancer Institute and the American Cancer Society are derelict in their duties to the people who support them."

Guinea Pigs in the War on Cancer

- The second half of the twentieth century saw medical progress moving at astonishing rates. Unfortunately, with that progress came record numbers of unethical experiments involving human subjects.

1963:   Dr. Chester M. Southam of Sloan Kettering injects live cancer cells into elderly indigent patients without their consent at Jewish Chronic Disease Hospital in Brooklyn.

- For example, in July 1963, after receiving funds from the U.S. Public Health Service and the American Cancer Society, researchers at the Jewish Chronic Disease Hospital sat in their offices and made their final selection regarding who would be injected with live human cancer cells. This was not some prison laboratory facility at Auschwitz; it was a New York hospital preparing to subject humans to Nazi-like experiments nearly twenty years after the defeat of Germany and three years after the election of John F. Kennedy, in what was described as the dawn of a new society.
- During the 1965 court case against the hospital [258 N.Y.S.2d 397], it must have seemed like déjà vu for Jews who'd seen it all before and sat horrified at the thought that it had happened at a Jewish hospital no less.
- The same type of cancer injections were also given to three hundred healthy women at Memorial Sloan-Kettering Cancer Center. According to Jay Katz, author of *Experimentation with Human Beings*, gynecology patients were injected with cancer without their knowledge in order to determine how the body would respond to an invasion of live cancer cells. During testimony, several doctors admitted that they believed the injected cells might cause cancer years later but injected them anyway. The reason for performing the experiment on nonconsenting subjects was obvious. Who in their right mind would be willing to consent to being injected with cancer?

    The testimony, at times chilling, was a reminder that such things were still very much possible. Patients with and without cancer had been chosen without their consent for a study to determine not only if foreign cancer cells would live longer in debilitated noncancer patients than in patients with cancer, but if cancer could actually be included by injection of live cells. Hospital administrators later tried to cover up the fact that many of the subjects were physically and mentally unable to give consent or that the consent had been fraudulently obtained after the injections were already administered. To add insult to injury, The American Cancer Society elected the study's principal investigator as the vice president of their organization.

Source: *In the Name of Science*.
- Several governmental agencies and private pharmaceutical companies conducted experimental testing on 400 African Americans. It was a notorious medical experiment in American history. It was called Tuskegee Syphilis Study from 1932 until 1972. The experiment ended only because a journalist exposed it.

    In the south, doctors were rendering African Black women infertile without their knowledge during other surgery. It was so common the procedure was called a Mississippi appendectomy.

The same was true in the north as recently as the 1970s when unnecessary hysterectomies were often performed on poor African American and Puerto Rican women.
Source: *New York Times*, 1/23/07. Book review by Denise Grady on *The Dark History of*

Medical Experimentation on Black Americans from Colonial Times to the Present. By Harriet A. Washington.

1964:   NIH Committee under Robert Livingston studies ethical issues in NIH [*National Institute of Health*] funded research and makes no recommendations for changes in regulations because "whatever NIH might do by way of designating a code or stipulating standards for acceptable clinical research would be likely to inhibit, delay, or distort the carrying out of clinical research . . ."

1966:   FDA issues regulations specifically defining requirements of informed consent at 21 CFR 130.37, later incorporated into 45 CFR 46.

1966:   NIH Office for Protection or Research Subjects [OPRR] was created and issues policies for the Protection of Human Subjects calling for establishment of independent review bodies later known as Institutional Review Boards.

6/16/1966: Henry K. Beecher publishes "Ethics and Clinical Research" in the *New England Journal of Medicine*, citing 22 examples of unethical research studies and suggesting that an ethical approach to human experimentation must include: (1) obtaining informed consent from the participant; (2) providing an intelligent, informed, conscientious, compassionate and responsible investigator; and (3) that the benefits gained from the research be commensurate with the risk.

1967:   British physician M. H. Pappworth publishes "Human Guinea Pigs," advising "No doctor has the right to choose martyrs for science or for the general good."

For many years scientists have been saying: "We must experiment on animals because we can't [may not] experiment on human beings." But we anti-vivisectionists have always said that EXPERIMENTS ON ANIMALS LEAD INEVITABLY TO EXPERIMENTS ON PEOPLE. NO HOSPITAL PATIENT TODAY IS ABSOLUTELY SAFE FROM EXPERIMENTATION.
Source: Hansard, House of Common Reports, 3rd Aug. 1971. http://www. animalvoices. org/ADAV/papworth.htm.

Beecher's 1996 article played a significant role in the implementation of federal rules governing the conduct of human experimentation in the USA, including a clear call for fully informed consent from research subjects.

Both Beecher's and Pappworth's efforts at reforming clinical research reflect the turbulent status of human experimentation in the decades after the development of the Nuremberg Code. In 1964, after years of deliberation and committee discussion, The World Medical Association, an international body representing physicians and researchers from countries around the world, adopted the Declaration of Helsinki which established new rules for human experimentation. This Declaration, in the words of Henry Beecher, offered "a more broadly useful instrument" than the "rigid set of legalistic demands" set out in the Nuremberg Code. The Declaration of Helsinki has been amended five times since its adoption. [For the most recent version, ratified in October 2000 in Edinburgh, Scotland, consult http://www.wma.net/e/policy/17-c_e.html.]

The publications of Beecher and Pappworth did not resolve all controversies in research ethics, as the periodic revisions of the Declaration of Helsinki and national regulations demonstrate. But they did prompt the public and the health professions to recognize that questionable research practices could be carried out, and even rewarded, in advanced, democratic states, and that careful attention to ethics should be part of every scientist's approach to research.

Dr. Henry Beecher was a graduate of Harvard Medical School. He was an anesthetist-in-chief at Massachusetts General Hospital. Harvard installed him in the world's first endowed professorship in anesthesiology.

British Physician Maureen H. Pappworth was a distinguished medical consultant.

Shame on You!

The AMA gave a wink and a nod and turned a blind eye during these horrific medical atrocities and on the other hand is very protective of their Machiavellian puppeteer, the pharmaceutical industry [Big Pharma] when vitamin therapies are discussed.

AMA, your name is *HYPOCRISY!*

"When you participate in clinical studies, you may be dealing with the dire consequences that come with them."

Controlled studies had been used periodically since the turn of the century, although one involving the citrus treatment of a group of British sailors for scurvy, a once fatal disease now known to be the result of a vitamin C deficiency, was first recorded in 1747. The AMA conducted a double-blind study in 1911, yet most of the studies were not blinded or randomized and didn't use placebos. [Recognition of the placebo as an effective control began in the 1930s, and the first actual trial of its effects was done in 1950.]

In Phase I studies, CDER [Center for Drug Evaluation & Research (part of FDA)] can impose a clinical hold [i.e., prohibit the study from proceeding or stop a trial that has started] for reasons of safety or because of a sponsor's failure to accurately disclose the risk of study to investigators. Although CDER routinely provides advice in such cases, investigators may choose to ignore any advice regarding the design of Phase I studies in areas other than patient safety.

What most volunteers aren't told is that the odds of surviving a Phase I trial are remote because the trial is not designed to deliver a cure or treatment but simply to test a "safe" dose—which means that patients not receiving the safe dose either become sicker or die from the treatment. The reason patients are not told this is because it would discourage people from signing up for Phase I trials. God forbid we inform those on whom we experiment that what we're really doing is ascertaining how much of a drug will kill them.
Source: *In the Name of Science*, Andrew Golisek.

- Many studies of drugs are used on high dosage to achieve a convincing therapeutic effect. However, in day-to-day practice the drug is often used in much lower dosage to avoid unwanted side effects.
- Phase I studies also evaluate drug metabolism, structure-activity relationships, and the mechanism of actions in humans. Since they're designed to test doses that have never been tested in humans, researchers have no idea how a particular patient will react to a drug at a given dose. Cancer drugs are especially sensitive, with a small dose not working at all and larger dose sometimes lethal. Sadly for the patient, it's pretty much guesswork at this point.
Source: http://bmi-com/c91/content/R.LL/84/2/124-9 References.

Phase II studies include the early controlled clinical studies conducted to obtain some preliminary data on the effectiveness of the drug for a particular indication or indications in patients with the disease or condition. This phase of testing also helps determine the common short-term side effects and risks associated with the drug. Phase II studies are typically well controlled, closely monitored, and conducted in a relatively small number of patients, usually involving several hundred people.

Phase III studies are expanded, controlled and uncontrolled trials. They are performed after preliminary evidence suggesting effectiveness if the drug has been obtained in Phase II, and are intended to gather the additional information about effectiveness and safety that is needed to evaluate the overall benefit-risk relationship of the drug. Phase III studies also provide an adequate basis for extrapolating the results to the general population and transmitting that information in the physician labeling. Phase III studies usually include several hundred to several thousand people.

In both Phase II and III, CDER can impose a clinical hold if a study is unsafe [as in Phase I] or if the protocol is clearly deficient in design in meeting its stated objectives [Phase II]. Great care is taken to ensure that this determination is not made in isolation, but rather reflects current scientific knowledge, agency experience with the design of clinical trials and experience with the class of drugs under investigation.

Accelerated development/review [*Federal Register*, April 15, 1992] is a highly specialized mechanism for speeding the development of drugs that promise significant benefit over existing therapy for serious life-threatening illnesses for which no therapy exists.

This process incorporates several novel elements aimed at ensuring that rapid development and review is balanced by safeguards to protect both the patients and the integrity of the regulatory process.

Accelerated development/review can be used under two special circumstances: when approval is based on evidence of the product's effect on a "surrogate end point" and when the FDA determines that safe use of a product depends on restricting its distribution or use. *A surrogate end point is a laboratory finding or physical sign that may not be a direct measurement of how a patient feels, functions, or survives but is still considered likely to predict therapeutic benefit for the patient.* The fundamental element of this process is that the manufacturers must continue testing after approval to demonstrate that the drug indeed provides therapeutic benefit to the patient. If not, the FDA can withdraw the product from the market more easily than usual.

Some additional perspectives on studies [an abstract].
Source: http://.bmi.com/c91/content/full/84/2/134-19 reference

- Positive results are therefore more widely distributed than negative ones.
- This imposes a severe bias on *meta-analysis*. If the data collected in a review are of sufficient quality and similar enough, they are summarized statistically in a *meta-analysis*, which generally provides a better overall estimate of a clinical effect on the results from individual studies.
    Source: http://www.cochrane.org/reviews/restruct.htm
    Author: Is this a stacked deck or what.

- The evaluation of published data can be based on different criteria. "Evidence based" means that the data are carefully analyzed according to strict rules, such as the *Cochrane criteria.* These results achieve a high degree of reliability. "*Science based*" describes the usual scientific approach, and a subjective component cannot be excluded. If the published data are not homogeneous, their evaluation may be "*consensus based*". In consensus conferences, "experts" form an opinion which is often taken for the truth. Both the selection of the experts and their approach in coming to their conclusions are subject to personal bias. Most if not all guidelines are consensus based. A source of error common to all three modes of analysis is the reduced probability of negative trials being published, particularly in English language journals.
    Author: An over-simplification example of reduced probability. You enroll patients in whom a pronounced difference is expected to obtain a positive result.
    Group A achieved good results; Group B did not. When you publish your results, you eliminate Group B. You have now tilted the outcome in your favor using reduced probability.

    - Hey, are these guys from Las Vegas?

- In studies financed by the pharmaceutical industry it seems realistic to assume the marketing aspects are not without influence on the study design.
- If the objective of the study is to obtain a positive result, the new treatment may not be compared with the best available alternative but rather with a conventional regime that is likely to be inferior.
- A positive result may be achieved by enrolling patients in whom a pronounced difference is expected. If a negative study is desired—for example, to demonstrate equivalence of two treatments such as Beta-blockers versus calcium channel blockers in chronic stable angina—small studies with a <u>limited power</u> are conducted, so that even large differences could not be detected.

    Author: Limited power in this sense means the number of patients in the study was too small.

    Author: And you thought only pro wrestling was fixed!

If I were a prosecutor [which I am not], I would indict the pharmaceutical industry's influence on physicians who coldly dismiss anecdotal evidence as worthless. I would charge the AMA with treating alternative medicine not be treated like a red-headed step-child. [That may not be politically correct but it makes my point.]

I would require all pharmaceutical companies after the first year of FDA approval of their new drug to:
- Report all pending litigation on the new drugs.
- Report additional side effects called in by patients using their drug that the manufacturer did not list.
- This must be done for 5 consecutive years or the FDA has a right to terminate the drug.
- If the drug is declared unsafe before that, the FDA will also terminate it.
- There should also be a commensurate compensatory damages served against the manufacturer.

Who is Watching the Watchers?

- Institutional review boards [IRBs] are used to ensure the rights and welfare of participants in clinical trials both before and during their trial participation. IRBs at hospitals and research institutions throughout the country make sure that participants are fully informed and have given their written consent before studies begin. IRBs are monitored by the FDA to protect and ensure the safety of participants in medical research.

    An IRB must be composed of no fewer than five experts and lay people with varying backgrounds to ensure a complete and adequate review of activities commonly conducted by research institutions. In addition to possessing the professional competence needed to review specific activities, an IRB must be able to ascertain the acceptability of applications and proposals in terms of institutional commitments and regulations, applicable law, standards of professional conduct and practice, and community attitudes. Therefore, IRBs must be composed of people whose concerns are in relevant areas.

However, according to a 1998 report by Health and Human Services Inspector General June Gibbs Brown, IRBs have some serious problems. The report claims that review boards review too much, too quickly, and with too little expertise; conduct minimal continuing review of approved research; ignore conflicts (professional, financial, etc.) that threatens their independence; and provide little training for investigators and board members.

- At the time they were established, IRBs were designated for a research world that no longer exists. Their intent was to monitor research conducted at a single site by a single investigator, primarily at a university or teaching hospital. Today, research is done at multi-sites, in trials across the country or around the world, sometimes involving hundreds of researchers and thousands of research subjects. The science has become so complex that many review board members don't have the expertise to question experiments; they depend on a "paper compliance" process rooted in trust, seldom if ever visit research sites, and rarely monitor actual conduct of research and informed consent procedures.

One recent phenomenon is the growing financial interest board members have in the research products being used in experiments. As long as IRB's consist of people directly affiliated with the research institute or who own stock in the company whose product is being tested, abuses will continue while reviewers look the other way and play dumb. The charade of monitoring scientists and informed consent is often just that, with human subjects the ultimate victims in a cruel game that in some cases has proven fatal.

- *Despite codes of conduct, ethical standards, and laws to ensure the presence of informed consent and understanding of an experiment, one of the biggest problems in research today, says Dr. Greg Koski, director of the Federal Office for Human Research Protections, is that the opposite is happening. "Too often individual research participants will enter a study believing that they are being treated when in fact they need to understand that if they are participating in research, treatment may not be part of that," Koski explains. Surprisingly, based on Dr. Koski's recent surveys, as many as 90 percent of current medical research projects have a problem with informed consent and as few as 30 percent of subjects could even explain what the experiments they were involved in were about.*

Thus, while we claim that human subjects are more protected against abuse than ever before, the reality is that unethical and often dangerous human medical experimentation continues to grow at an alarming rate.

Source: *In the Name of Science.* Andrew Golisek.

- Because of these limitations, most of our therapeutic decisions are not entirely the result of evidence-based medicine. In daily routine practice, empirical criteria—including psychological, social, economic, medical, and technical factors—are at least equally important. The choice of treatment should be tailored to each patient and be based on both objective and subjective criteria—that is, evidence-based and experience-based medicine.
- Undoubtedly evidence-based medicine is the gold standard for modern medicine. The results, however, should be applied in patient care with careful reflection. Otherwise evidence-based medicine may acquire the same status for the doctor as a lamp post for a drunk: it gives more support than enlightenment.

Paul's Trials

Webster says: "trial: a try-out or experiment to test quality or usefulness."

You're probably asking yourself, why are Paul's trials in this chapter? I'll give you two good reasons:

1. If I don't qualify as an experimental lab rat after you have read Dr. Feel Good's "lowering my cholesterol to 99" and wanting it lower by doubling up on my statin doses, I don't know who would.
2. I wrote the book.

I not only needed an internist thanks to Dr. Phil [*no, not the one on TV*], I also needed a cardiologist.

Don't you hate it when doctors don't work out and upset your life.

You don't have to answer. It's rhetorical.

Dr. Randy, cardiologist a/k/a switchboard operator and is one of those prescription writers. I'll never forget him.

My first visit, I brought [*typed, I want you to know and in chronological order yet*]:
o Medical diagnoses
o List of medications and dosage strengths
o Exercise routine
o My vitamins regime
o All my medical and latest tests
o My echocardiogram and stress test.

The receptionist took my "documents" and told me to go into the exam room. [*You know the drill. Go into a freezing exam room. Strip, put on the latest "Prada" fashion with the draft in the back*]. "The doctor will be in momentarily." [*Was she kidding? It seemed like dog years.*] Momentarily, I use the word in dog years, in came Dr. Randy. Before I could talk,

36

he grabbed the phone on the wall without even an "Excuse me," he started talking to a call-in patient.

- I wasn't interested in how Ms. M. was reacting to her angina meds. [*That took five minutes. I was freezing.*]
- Nor was I interested in Mr. W's gas and flatulence that his meds caused. [*I am guessing again: It seemed like 6 minutes.*]

His office assistant walked in while he was on the phone and said he was wanted at the Glen Cove Hospital.

I said, "Dr. R., before you run, I need 6 prescriptions with 3 refills each." [*Who knows when I'll see him again!*]

He said, "Tell my assistant what you want. I'll sign them after my next phone call."

He signed my prescriptions on the way out the door and told me to book another appointment.

On my second appointment, I was determined to get his opinion of my "documents" and provide a medical strategy.

- I waited in exam room #1 [*in my Prada*]. In he strode.
- I said, "Dr. R., what type of medical strategy are we ever going to use?" He called me Paul [*that relaxed me*]. "We will start with a stress test." [*I guess the dog ate my documents; you must be kidding!*].
- I said, "Dr. R., you're holding in your hand my latest stress test results. I had a stress test 4 weeks ago." [*You guessed it. The deer-in-the-headlights look!*]

The next few minutes were not pretty.

I never saw Dr. Randy again. *I thought this would benefit both of us.*

Nobody is perfect! Hey, he gets a ten on prescription writing and, don't forget, I got 3 refills. *He gets a two on switchboard.*

I decided to take a little R & R looking for another cardiologist instead of using "Mapquest." After all, I had 4 months of prescriptions to tide me over.

Someone who will remain nameless recommended an internist who was in my next zip code.

Enter Dr. William, Internist a/k/a Dr. Kevorkian.

- Again I handed in my typed documents. [*I had copies. Somehow I knew my doctor quest would be episodic.*]

o They had a great reception area: music, a small waterfall; a pitcher of fresh water with lemons.
o The pièce de resistance with a fully equipped gym you could see through a picture window. I thought I reached my medical Mecca [*which would be short-lived.*]
o I went to exam room #2 [*I was moving up in the medical world*], got into my Prada with the rear vent, and waited.
o In came an assistant to:
  - draw blood. It took 4 attempts. [*The next day I looked like somebody hit me in the arm with a baseball bat. The hematoma was a 5" diameter.*]
  - give me a metabolism test. [*The doctor never discussed the results.*]
  - give me a bone density test. [*The doctor never discussed the results of this test either. I cut him off at the pass. – I got copies at my next appointment at the front desk.*]
o When Dr. W came in, he was accompanied by an intern from LIJ who [*as I was told by Dr. W*] was to be an observer. When he read my documents, he said he thought the lab work I brought in was excellent.
o He thought the vitamin list looked good. – *I felt he only had a nodding acquaintance with vitamins.* He called my aortic valve "tight." I think that's medical slang for my aortic stenosis. He recommended – *since he saw I was into vitamins* – to read Dr. Dean Ornish's book on *How to Reverse Arterio-Sclerosis.* He told me to pay particular attention to the chapter on stress. Last but far from least, he told me, after looking at my echocardiogram – *and I'll never forget this* – "If I were a betting man, which I am not, they will be replacing your aortic valve within 2 years." That was three years ago, and I am still asymptomatic. I told him he made my day, which ended my first experience with Dr. Kevorkian.

My second visit with Dr. William a/k/a Dr. K. was about 10 days later.

o In strode Dr. K. with an intern observer. He was very jovial. He said,
o my labs were really great [*improved over the ones I brought him on my first visit, which were 4 weeks old*].
o He had looked over my echocardiogram and said my heart was in great shape. [*Was he being nice to me because he was feeling contrite for his Gestapo-style psychology he used on me at my last visit?*].
o He asked if I read Dr. Ornish's book, especially the chapter on stress. [*I no sooner replied yes when he dropped a stress grenade on me; then, the coup de grace Gestapo-style psychology.*]
o He said [*and I'll never forget this either*], "Your aortic valve is so tight that if you're out on a course playing golf and you go down, they will never bring you around with C.P.R. I said, that's very reassuring." That's the last I saw of him.

As a footnote: I don't know if he had a consultation room because I never saw it. Was I lucky or what?

I must draw to these type of doctors like a moth to a flame. A friend at the club who knew I was into vitamins because I told him to take glucosamine/chondrohtin for his knee [*he worshiped me for that advice*] he said he just started to see a new cardiologist [who was also, he thought (*but I found out better)* into vitamins]. I said, "you're playing my song" and called the next day for an appointment.

My first pro-forma visit:
- I gave the receptionist my documents.
- Was sent to exam room A. [*Did this mean I finally made it?*]
- Put on my Prada with the vent and got goose bumps waiting for my new medical discovery. I was beginning to feel like a medical explorer.
- In strode [*they all stride*] Dr. F. He was all business and as warm as the frigid room temperature.
- He read my documents or at least it appeared that he did.
- We got down to brass tacks; he scheduled, for my second visit:
  o an echo cardiogram
  o a stress test
  o a lower arterial examination
  o plus blood work. [[I got a prescription to go to a private lab. My arm was still black and blue from Dr. Kevorkian's assistant.]

My second visit:
  o again the Prada
  o a stress test exam with
  o an echocardiogram
  o a lower arterial examination.

*A footnote: Whenever you go into his office, you give the following information:
  o List of meds you use
  o Exercise you are doing
  o Drinking, smoking etc., etc.

My third visit:
  o Again the Prada with the vent and the goose bumps. [*The exam room was like a meat locker.*]
  o In strode Dr. F. [*What else?*]
    [*I was relaxed. I knew at this point which was 6 weeks after my tests (yes, I had copies) everything was fine, in fact my EF (ejection factor) went up to 63%*]. He asked what type of exercise I was doing and I told him it was on the form he was holding in his hand that I filled out at reception. [*Why?*]
  o He said he wanted me to take an angiogram at St. Francis. [*Brace yourself, here comes the Gestapo-style!*]
  o He said, had I ever heard of Jim Kick, the marathon runner, who dropped dead of a heart attack while running. I replied, or course I did. What was his point?
  o He said, "he was asymptomatic. So are you. You could drop dead at any time [*like he* did] while you're riding your bike. [*In case you forgot, at the time I was riding 8 miles [every day]. Since then I ride 8 miles and row 1 miles for a total of 9 miles.*]

    o I told him no. But finally agreed to a new non-invasive type angiogram. [*It was later cancelled the following week, when he finally found in my documents my Calcium Coronary score test. The test he wanted me to take would be invalid because of the excessive calcification in my heart. He never told me why he canceled the test. It was my sense that he had never read up on all the tests in my documents. If he had, he would have realized that fact.*]

My 4th visit [*so far, this is a record for me with new doctors*] was the day after he canceled my non-invasive angiogram,
    o He said he wanted me to go to St. Francis for a stress test. [*I said no.*]
    o He wanted to increase my Lipitor from 20 mg to 40 mg. [He had taken me off Zetia.] *My HDL was 99. My triglycerides was 70, my HDL was 45, and my LDL was 40.*
    o I told him of the research I did on Dr. David L. Tirschell of Harborview Medical Center in Seattle who conducted a study indicating people with a cholesterol under 180 could have hemorrhagic strokes. *He said the tests were skewed and were not reliable.*
    o He also did not know about the rule of the sixes regarding doubling my dose of statins. *By doubling, you only get a 6% reduction. In my case, he would lower from 40 to 38.60.* [*I had no intention of being his lab rat.*]
    o I told him, no way.
    o He then applied his Gestapo-type psychology. A real coup de grace.
    o He said [*another memorable medical statement I will never forget*].
       - "If you had been seeing another cardiologist, you would have had your aortic valve replaced by now."
       - "You would have had your carotid artery repaired."
    o I just looked at him, said "you made my day," and walked out. *If you don't think he was experimenting on me, I rest my case.*

Folks, you can't make this up. It's pretty pathetic. So it shouldn't be a total loss, if I could get a sponsor, I could do at least 4 weeks on summer TV. I would call it, "Who's your Doctor?" Hell, I already auditioned part of my cast.

- Dr. Phil [*not the one on TV, but my original internist*], a/k/a What's happening? Or don't confuse me with medical terms.
- Dr. Randy, a/k/a Cordon Bleu prescription writer and part-time switchboard operator.
- Dr. William, a/k/a Dr. Kevorkian.
- Dr. F, a/k/a Dr. Feel Good.

Hey, I got a great idea for a sponsor:

- Lipitor and the AMA. All I need is an agent.
- Oh. I forgot to mention, none of the above even broached suggesting a nutritional, exercise and prescriptions strategy, with the exception of Dr. Sinatra and my

present medical doctor [*record holder – it's been 18 months*], cardiologist, Dr. Frederick Vagnini of Garden City, New York.

Note: This chapter or any other chapter in this book is not meant to dispense medical advice or strategies for your health care. It is meant to raise your awareness to be pro-active to other health options which should be discussed with your health care professional.

CHAPTER 5

All is not Lost

Don't panic! Remember, you're not on the *Titanic*.

For readers who missed the movie and you history buffs:

Titanic Facts: The unsinkable *Titanic* was built in Belfast, Ireland. It sunk on April 14, 1912, on its maiden voyage, in approx. 3 hours, 1,000 miles due East of Boston. It was 882 feet long. It was approx. 11 stories high; weighed over 46,000 tons. It was built at a cost of $400,000.00. Today, it would cost an estimated $7,500,000.00. Of the 2,228 crew and passengers on board, there were only 705 survivors.

All is Really Not Lost *[because you were not on the Titanic]*

During my research for this book I was struck by the similarity Big Pharma has to the HYDRA. [For all of you who fell asleep during Greek mythology – he was the monster with nine heads; when one head was struck off by Hercules, it was replaced by two new ones.]

In spite of all of the **heads** of Big Pharma, influencing:
- The Congress and Senate in Washington, DC,
- The FDA,
- The AMA,
- Grants distorting clinical studies,
- Grants to medical schools influencing curriculums,
- The media bias on nutritional supplements we see on T.V. and read in magazines and the newspaper daily,

there are some outstanding individual physicians and one medical organization I know of who still honor the Hippocratic Oath. [The two following paragraphs make my point.]

> I will apply, for the benefit of the sick, all measures [that] are required, avoiding those twin traps of overtreatment and therapeutic nihilism.

> I will remember that there is art to medicine as well as science, and that warmth, sympathy, and understanding may outweigh the surgeon's knife or the chemist's drug.

Two of these I have mentioned in this book [notwithstanding Dr. Stephen Sinatra and Dr. Frederick Vagnini]:

- Dr. Jerome D. Kassierer [see Chapter III] in his statement to the Ways & Means Committee, where he said it all.
- Dr. Ajal R. Singh of India – in this chapter, who also has picked up the gauntlet.

- Dr. Carolyn Dean [see Chapter V. Statins]
- The National Center for Complementary and Alternative Medicine [NCCAM].

Let's have a standing round of applause for this physician from India, Ajal R. Singh, founder of Mens Sana Research Foundation, Mumbai, India.

Abstract from his Academia-Industry Symposium 2005-2006:
- Where is medicine heading? Pointers and directions from recent law suits against the pharmaceutical industry [Big Pharma].
- Companies like Glaxo-SmithKline, Bayer, Bristol-Myers Squibb, AstraZeneca, Schering-Plough, Abbott Labs, TAP Pharmaceuticals, Wyeth and Merck have paid millions of dollars each as compensation in the last few years. The financial condition of many pharmaceutical majors is not buoyant either. Price deflation, increased random spending, and litigation costs are the main reasons. In the future, the messy lawsuit situations would no longer be restricted to industry. It would involve academia and practicing doctors as well. Indian pharma industry captains, who were busy raking in the profits at present, would also come under the scanner. If nothing else, it means industry and docs will have to sit down and do some soul searching.
- Both short- and long-term measures will have to be put into place. Short-term measures involve reduction in (1) pharma spending over junkets and trinkets; (2) hype over 'me too' drugs; (3) manipulation of drug trials; (4) getting pliant researchers into drug trials; (5) manipulation of journal editors to publish positive findings about their drug trials and launches; (6) and for Indian Pharma to conduct their own unbiased clinical trial of the latest drug projected as a blockbuster in the West, before pumping in their millions.

Well, you might ask: why are we ringing these alarm bells?
- It's because the wants [not needs] of the medical man have multiplied beyond imagination. Each one of them wants to be pampered by the pharmaceuticals. Conferences have to be in *Five Star* hotels, and delegates must be housed in *Five Stars* too; they must travel by air, and must be shown around the place. Complementary. The odd gift will no longer do. Expensive holidays, foreign trips, personal accessories must be lavishly thrown in to pamper the man of medicine. And he is like a man-eater. Having once tasted the blood of pampering, he will not settle for anything less.
- The cost of organizing conferences is no longer even possible on delegate fees. The sponsors have ensured that they can never be done away with. The plastic smiles and courtesies in looking after delegates, who expect everything on the house and snide at the way medicine is gravitating. Happy at the way medicine is playing itself completely into the hands of commerce.
- The sponsorship must translate into prescriptions. First gentle and then more insistent reminders make their way into conversation. Well, if the healing man feels irked, it's absolutely on purpose. It pays to be loyal, to write the latest drugs hyped, to speak well of the new drug launch at sponsored CMEs, workshops, conferences, etc. Never mind the doc concerned is really not convinced.

- Unfortunately, a few monkey wrenches in the works have been placed lately. Patients expect drugs to work beyond placebo effect. Patients expect docs to be clean. Patients expect docs not to get involved in a nexus with pharmaceuticals.
- The whole brunt of this movement is borne by guess who—that hapless consumer, the patient waiting patiently outside the clinic door.
- Probably, he had rightly been called a patient. He has been patient enough.
- Glaxo-SmithKline, Bayer, Pfizer, Bristol-Myers Squibb, AstraZeneca, Schering-Plough, Abbott Labs, TAP Pharmaceuticals, Wyeth, Merck. None of them small names. All of them have paid millions of dollars as compensation in the last few years.

Glaxo SmithKline agreed to pay U.S. $2.5 million for charges that it suppressed findings that showed its antidepressant, Paxil, was harmful in children. It paid $75 million for allegedly overcharging patients and insurers for its anti-inflammatory drug, Relafen. It also agreed to pay US $ 92 million to end law suits over Augmentin, its antibiotic. Bayer settled over 2,000 cases brought up against the drug Baycol, at a cost of US $ 800 million. Pfizer paid US $ 430 million to settle claims against off-label use of its drug, Neurotin. It is being sued at present by consumer groups claiming that the company misleadingly marketed its blockbuster cholesterol-lowering drug, Lipitor [*Datamonitor Newswire*, 30 Sept. 2005]. Bristol-Myers Squibb promised to pay US $ 300 million to fend off a lawsuit by its own shareholders. In 2003, Astra Zeneca settled criminal fraud charges of US $ 355 million in a case dealing with its drug Zoladex [Peterson, 2003]. On July 14, 2004, Schering-Plough pleaded guilty of and was fined US $ 350 million in part for providing 'educational grants' to physicians, which were more appropriately called 'kickbacks' by the prosecutors [Harris, 16 July, 2004b]. It faces an ongoing investigation whether or not it used sham consulting arrangements and clinical trials to remunerate doctors for writing its hepatitis drug, Antron A [Harris, 27 June, 2004a]. TAP Pharmaceuticals entered into a settlement and paid US $ 290 million in criminal fines, plus US § 585 million in civil penalties, out of which US $ 100 million went to whistle blowers [*United States v. TAP Pharmaceuticals*, Dec. 14, 2001]. It continues to face further lawsuits by insurers and patients for unnecessary and costly services. All related to the way it used urologists to promote its Lupron, a potent gonadotropin-releasing hormone used in treating prostate cancer. Wyeth has had a US $ 1 billion verdict against it for its Pondlimin, an anti-obesity drug. The most recent Vioxx catastrophe is likely to result in a US $ 10-15 billion litigation bill [Horton, 2004b] for the company involved, Merck, and probably cripple both its financial status as well as its reputation beyond repair.*
> [*He, of course, is referring to Jerome Kassierer's statement to the House of Representative's Ways and Means Committee, Subcommittee on Health.]

On Our side of the Ocean, educational programs are in place in NYS [as in other states] by Attorney General Consumer Prescriber Education Gant Program.

Money for the educational programs comes from a $430 million dollar settlement that resolved charges that pharmaceutical grant Pfizer, Inc. illegally paid doctors to prescribe its drug Neurontin for uses that had not been approved by the U.S. Food & Drug Administration.

- Medical schools in several states are strengthening programs that warn doctors and students not to be dazzled by drug company marketing practices.

- The pharmaceutical industry [Big Pharma] spends billions of dollars a year on advertising and lavish sales pitches to doctors, prompting concerns that slick promotion is unduly influencing how medications get prescribed.
- The Mount Sinai School of Medicine announced that it would use a $400,000 grant from that settlement to remind doctors to question sophisticated sales presentations and rely on solid science when deciding which medications to give patients.
- "We want to appeal to physicians' natural skepticism," said Dr. Ethan Halm, an associate professor of medicine and health policy at Mount Sinai.
- The program is one of five receiving $1.9 million from the Attorney General Consumer and Prescriber Education Grant Program, which has awarded $11 million to 28 institutions interested in cautioning health care workers about pharmaceutical sales techniques.

Source: http://www.commercialalert.org/news/archive/2006/11/medical-schools train-doctors-to-resist ma...

<u>Don't look now but I think the Cavalry is Coming.
It's called NCCAM – National Center for
Complementary and Alternative Medicine.</u>

The National Center for Complementary and Alternative Medicine [NCCAM] is the Federal Government's lead agency for scientific research on complementary and alternative medicine [CAM]. They are 1 of the 27 institutes and centers that make up the National Institutes of Health [NIH] within the U.S. Department of Health and Human Services.

CAM is a group of diverse medical and health care systems, practices, and products that are not presently considered to be part of conventional medicine. Complementary medicine is used together with conventional medicine, and alternative medicine is used in place of conventional medicine. Conventional medicine is medicine as practiced by holders of M.D. [medical doctor] or D.O. [doctor of osteopathy] degrees and by their allied health professionals, such as physical therapists, psychologists, and registered nurses. Some health care providers practice both CAM and conventional medicine.

The list of practices that are considered CAM changes continually, as those therapies that are proven to be safe and effective become adopted into conventional health care and as new approaches to health care emerge.

The mission of NCCAM is to:
- Explore complementary and alternative healing practices in the context of rigorous science.
- Train complementary and alternative medicine researchers.
- Disseminate authoritative information to the public and professionals.

NCCMA sponsors and conducts research using scientific methods and advanced technologies to study CAM. CAM is a group of diverse medical and health care systems, practices, and products that are not presently considered to be part of conventional medicine.

- NCCAM has four primary areas of focus:
  1. *Advancing scientific research.*
     They have funded more than 1,200 research projects at scientific institutions across the United States and around the world.
  2. *Training CAM researchers*
     They support training for new researchers as well as encourage experienced researchers to study CAM.
  3. *Sharing news and information*
     They provide timely and accurate information about CAM research in many ways, such as through their Web site, our information clearinghouse, fact sheets, Distinguished Lecture Series, continuing medical education programs, and publication databases.
  4. *Supporting integration of proven CAM therapies*
     Their research helps the public and health professionals understand which CAM therapies have been proven to be safe and effective.

NCCAM Clearinghouse
Get answers to your questions about complementary and alternative medicine or NCCAM.

Toll-free: 1-888-644-6226; Hrs.: M/F 8:30 a.m. – 5:00 p.m. EST
International: 301-519-3153
TTY [for deaf or hard-of-hearing callers]: 1-866-464-3615

E-mail: info@nccam.nih.gov
Web site: mccam.nih.gov
Address: NCCAM Clearinghouse, P.O. Box 7923, Gaithersburg, MD 20898-7923

Fax: 1-866-464-3616
Fax-on-Demand Service: 1-888-644-6226

Source: http://nccam.nih.gov/camonpubmed/background.htm

Note: This chapter or any other chapter in this book is not meant to dispense medical advice or strategies for your health care. It is meant to raise your awareness to be pro-active to other health options which should be discussed with your health care professional.

CHAPTER 6

Statins and Some Other Drugs

For those of you that have elevated triglycerides and homocysteine levels, statins have no effect at all and are not very effective, if at all, in raising HDL.

I would like to share with you an abstract of a very well study sponsored by Big Pharma, in this case, Pfizer.

Intensive Cholesterol Lowering with Atorvastatin Halts Progression of Heart Disease, Cleveland-Led Study Shows "REVERSAL" Trial Results to be published March 3, 2004 in JAMA.

- The first head-to-head comparison <u>of two popular cholesterol-lowering medications</u> showed that only one of the statins successfully stopped the progression of heart disease. The Cleveland Clinic-led research also found that people's cholesterol levels had to be cut to much lower levels than national guidelines currently recommend to achieve this result.
- The REVERSAL TRIAL DIRECTED BY Cleveland Clinic cardiologist Steven Nissen, M.D., <u>compared the highest doses available at the time of two popular statin drugs,</u> pravastatin and atorvastatin. Both medications work to block the liver's ability to produce harmful cholesterol, which can clog coronary arteries. Complete trial results will be published March 3, in the *Journal of the American Medical Association.*

Their study started approximately 9/03/2003. At that time, among other popular statins, in addition to cited pravastatin [Pravachol] and atorvastatin [Lipitor], there were Rosuvastatin [Crestor], and simvastatin [Zocor]. I think, not using the brand names but the generic names causes further confusion [at least in my case] in trying to understand the study. I think this was by design to confuse the lay person reading this on a website.

- "When we analyze the results of REVERSAL, we realize that we had found an approach to coronary disease treatment that could literally stop heart disease in its tracks," Dr. Nissen said. "Additional research must be done to verify our conclusions, but this is potentially life-altering news for millions of people suffering from heart disease."

The REVERSAL study randomly split 502 patients into equal-sized groups to receive either 40-mg doses of pravastatin or 80-mg doses of atorvastatin for 18 months of treatment. The progression of their heart disease was measured using intravascular ultrasound, which allows scientists to see plaque buildup in coronary arteries over time.

<u>"The results were striking," Dr. Nissen said, "demonstrating a complete halting of coronary disease progression in the atorvastatin-treated patients and continued progression of disease in the pravastatin-treated group."</u>

Author's comparison of the two statins' effectiveness used in the study and two other popular cholesterol-lowering statins (Crestor and Zocor) that they implied were not available at the time of the study.

Generic Name		Brand Name	Average Expected LDL Reduction
Atorvastatin	80 mg	Lipitor	46% - 51%
Pravastatin	40 mg	Pravachol	26% - 34%
Resuvastatin	40 mg	Crestor	55% - 60%*
Simvastatin	40 mg	Zocor	35% - 45%*

*LDL reductions from other studies.

Author: If he was being unbiased, he should have presented the statins in this manner and then selected Crestor in his study. But, as you know, he used the least effective of the three to further prove his biased study.

- The more intensively treated atorvastatin patients reached an LDL-C level [the bad cholesterol] of 79 milligrams per deciliter [mg/dL] while the more moderately treated pravastatin patients achieved an LDL-C of 110 mg/dL].

Author: I feel Dr. Nissen, by design, did not use the transparency understandable to the lay person. He should have given base lines at the study's inception [e.g., cholesterol ____, triglycerides _____, HDL _____, LDL _____, HDL/LDL ratio _____ before as complete baselines for the study using 80 mg/dL of Lipitor, and not only showing the one baseline of LDL.

Dr. Feel Good [before I escaped] had me on 20 mg Lipitor which he wanted to double to 40 mg. My labs were cholesterol 99, triglycerides 70, HDL 45m LDL 40, Ratio 2.2.

In addition to the Lipitor, I was also using a fiber product named Pro-Fibe, in addition to my vitamin regimen. I stopped the Pro-Fibe for 10 weeks to try to raise my cholesterol. My new labs: cholesterol 131, triglycerides 80, HDL 62, LDL 53, Ratio 2.1. The below-average risk of cholesterol/HDL ratio is below 4.2.

- The pravastatin-treated patients experienced a 2.7 percent increase in the volume of atherosclerotic plaque, while the atorvastatin-treated patients showed a 0.4 percent decrease. The 0.4 percent decrease in plaque was statistically "no change" from baseline, meaning that **no** progression had occurred in the atorvastatin-treated group. Another important finding of REVERSAL was the effect of atorvastatin and pravastatin on C-reactive protein [CRP], an important measure of artery inflammation linked to an increased risk of heart attack. In the REVERSAL study, patients treated with pravastatin showed a 5.2-percent reduction in CRP, while those treated with atorvastatin showed a 36.4-percent decrease.

Patients who reached a low LDL-level on pravastatin continued to show disease progression. For any degree of reduction of cholesterol achieved during treatment, the progression rate was slower if the patient reached that cholesterol level by taking atorvastatin. <u>The REVERSAL authors suggest that the greater reduction in CRP may partially explain the better results observed in the atorvastatin-treated patients.</u>

The study was funded by Pfizer, maker of atorvastatin [Lipitor], but was conducted independently by The Cleveland Clinic Cardiovascular Coordinating Center. All measurements were performed by the intravascular Ultrasound Core Laboratory at The Cleveland Clinic, and the manuscript generated by Dr. Nissen and co-authors.

http://www.clevelandclinic.org/heartcenter/pub/news/archive/2004,reversal5_2asp.

Author: My final comments on Dr. Nissen's format in presenting the conclusions to his Reversal Study:

This would be a more comprehensive and understandable format:

	Lowered LDL	Decrease Plaque	Increase Plaque	Decrease CRP
Atorvastatin [LIPITOR] 80 mg	to 79%	.04%	0	36.4%
Pravastatin [PRAVACHOL] 40 mg	to 110%	0	2.7%	5.2%

Author: It is general knowledge in the medical field, the higher dosage usually leads to more effectiveness and, of course, exposes you to greater danger of side effects.

Unfortunately, because he did not give me baselines for the other cholesterol values, you can't get a full impact of my lower dosage with the addition of my vitamins' and nutritional supplements' effect, except the comparison of Lipitor 80 mg lowered it to 79, whereas my strategy with only 20 mg of Lipitor [putting me at lower risk for side effects] at 53 is a much better place to stop plaque formation and perhaps reverse it.

There are over 130 side effects of statins that have been reported by statin manufacturers.

Author: Using the lowest possible dose of drugs with vitamins and nutritional supplements to achieve the best possible results is the best of both worlds.

I feel you have not unnecessarily exposed yourself to possible horrific side-effects.

The progression of my aortic valve and carotid artery stenosis had become life threatening to me. I had to [so to speak] find something to plug the dike, and that was statin drugs.

I am limiting my examples to these statin drugs I have personally used.

- ZETIA is a medicine used to lower levels of total cholesterol and LDL [bad] cholesterol in the blood. It is used for patients who cannot control their cholesterol levels by diet alone. It can be used by itself or with other medicines to treat high cholesterol. You should stay on a cholesterol-lowering diet while taking this medicine. [*My research could not find expected LDL reduction for Zetia.*]
ZETIA works to reduce the amount of cholesterol your body absorbs. ZETIA does not help you to lose weight.
  - If you have active liver disease, do not take ZETIA while taking cholesterol-lowering medicines called statins.
  - If you are pregnant or breast-feeding, do not take ZETIA while taking a statin.
  - Keep taking ZETIA unless your doctor tells you to stop. It is important that you keep taking ZETIA even if you do not feel sick.
See your doctor regularly to check your cholesterol level and to check for side effects. Your doctor may do blood tests to check your liver before you start taking ZETIA or a statin drug, and during treatment.

What are the possible side effects of ZETIA?

In clinical studies patients reported few side effects while taking ZETIA. These included stomach pain and feeling tired.
Very rarely, patients have experienced severe muscle problems while taking ZETIA, usually when ZETIA was added to a statin drug. If you experience unexplained muscle pain, tenderness, or weakness while taking Zetia, contact your doctor immediately. You need to do this promptly, because on rare occasions, these muscle problems can be serious, with muscle breakdown resulting in kidney damage. Additionally, the following side effects have been reported in general use: allergic reactions [which may require treatment right away] including swelling of the face, lips, tongue, and/or throat that may cause difficulty in breathing or swallowing, rash, and hives; joint pain; muscle aches; alterations in some laboratory blood tests; liver problems; inflammation of the pancreas; nausea; gallstones; and inflammation of the gallbladder.

Source: Merck/Schering-Plough Pharmaceuticals

What is LIPITOR? [I had Dr. Randy prescribe that for me because Zetia was not accomplishing what I was hoping for.]
- LIPITOR is a prescription medicine that lowers cholesterol in your blood. It lowers the LDL-C ["bad" cholesterol] in your blood. It can raise your HDL-C ["good" cholesterol] as well. LIPITOR is for adults and children over 10 whose cholesterol does not come down enough with exercise and a low-fat diet alone.
LIPITOR can lower the risk for heart attack or stroke in patients who have risk factors for heart disease such as:
  - age, smoking, high blood pressure, low HDL-C, heart disease in the family, or
  - diabetes with risk factor such as eye problems, kidney problems, smoking, or high blood pressure.

What are the Possible Side Effects of LIPITOR?

- **LIPITOR can cause serious side effects. These side effects have happened only to a small number of people. Your doctor can monitor you for them. These side effects usually go away if your dose is lowered or LIPITOR is stopped. These serious side effects include:**
  - **Muscle problems.** LIPITOR can lead to serious muscle problems that can lead to kidney problems, including kidney failure. You have a higher chance of muscle problems if you are taking certain other medicines with LIPITOR.
  - **Liver problems.** LIPITOR can cause liver problems. Your doctor may do blood tests to check your liver before you start taking LIPITOR, and while you take it.

  Source [abstracted]: Pfizer Pharmaceuticals

VYTORIN

I had Dr. Vagnini prescribe Vytorin 10/20 replacing the Lipitor 20 mg I had been taking. I was hoping that with the Vytorin and the pro Fibe to get closer to the results Dr. Nissen was getting in the reversal study using 80 mg of Lipitor [without taking that strength statin] which, I felt, could have disastrous side effects.

New drug to lower cholesterol on way

TRENTON – Vytorin, the first pill to lower cholesterol in two ways, will likely hit pharmacy shelves within weeks, the makers said recently as they promised heavy marketing and discounted prices to battle the top-selling competition.

A joint venture between pharmaceutical companies Merck & Co. and Schering-Plough Corp. late Friday won U.S. Food & Drug Administration approval for Vytorin as a supplement to dieting – an approval crucial for both companies.

Schering-Plough, of Kenilworth, N.J. has been struggling through four straight losing quarters, falling sales because of increased competition and a host of legal and regulatory problems. Whitehouse Station, N.J.-based Merck reported flat profits last quarter, saw four promising drugs fail in mid- to late-stage testing last year and is facing generic competition for Zocor, its biggest seller, in 2006.

During conference calls with industry analysts and reporters yesterday, company officials said Vytorin does a better job of lowering LDL, or so-called bad cholesterol, than competitor Pfizer Inc.'s top-selling Lipitor or Merck's Zocor, the No. 2 cholesterol drug in the $15 billion U.S. market.

"We believe Vytorin will be a very strong competitor in the United States," said Adam Schechter, vice president and general manager of the joint venture, Merck/Schering-Plough Pharmaceuticals.

The new drug is likely to benefit from new national guidelines calling for more aggressive cholesterol-lowering, with recommendations that patients at highest risk of heart attack and stroke get their LDL level below 100.

Vytorin combines Zocor, at one of four different doses, with 10 milligrams of Zetia, the first cholesterol drug produced by the joint venture.

"Vytorin is the first and only product approved to treat the two sources of cholesterol in one pill," said Dr. Rick Veltri, group vice president of worldwide clinical development for Schering-Plough Research Institute.

Schechter said the joint venture hopes to officially launch the new drug before Labor Day.

Vytorin will have a wholesale price of $2.34 for each of its four doses – 10 milligrams of Zocor combined with 10, 20, 40 or 80 milligrams of Zetia.

By comparison, Pfizer's Lipitor sells for $2.10 wholesale for a 10-milligram pill and $3 for an 80-milligram pill. Zocor sells for $2.20 for a 10-milligram pill and $3.83 for the three higher doses.

Zetia sells for $2.16 per pill.

Source: Newsday, Tuesday July 27, 2004. [I started Vytorin 7/2005.]

STATIN CHOICES TO LOWER LDL < 30%

CR Best Buy	Generic Name with Dose Per Day	Brand Name	Average Monthly Cost	Average Expected LDL Reduction	Reduces the Risk of Heart Attack?
	Atorvastatin				Yes
	Atorvastatin 10 mg	Lipitor	$ 90	34% - 38%	
	Atorvastatin 20 mg	Lipitor	$129	42% - 46%	
	Atorvastatin 40 mg	Lipitor	$129	47% - 51%	
	Atorvastatin 80 mg	Lipitor	$128	46% - 54%	
	Ezetimibe/simvastatin 10 mg/10 mg	Vytorin	$195	45%	
	Ezetimibe/simvastatin 10 mg/20 mg	Vytorin	$104	52%	
	Ezetimibe/simvastatin 10 mg/40 mg	Vytorin	$104	55%	
	Ezetimibe/simvastatin 10 mg/80 mg	Vytorin	$103	60%	

Drug Reactions Underreported

The number of adverse drug reactions is growing more than twice as fast as the number of prescriptions being filled in the US. From 1994 to 2003, the number of bad drug reactions reported jumped 145% while the number of prescriptions filled increased 59%.

The FDA estimates that about 390,000 adverse reactions will be reported this year. Yet the FDA cautions that the actual number is likely to be between 10 and 100 times higher because of under-reporting.

The issue of drug reaction and monitoring is a simple case of numbers. Before the FDA approves a drug safe for sale, it's tested on a few thousand people. It's enough of a sample to find big and obvious side effects, the kind that hit maybe one out of every 100 users.

When drugs are sold commercially and used by millions of patients, rare side effects can show up, some with deadly consequences. A rare side effect that would hurt maybe one person in 10,000 wouldn't show up in the initial study, but it would in the mass marketplace.

[*Source:* www.jsonline.com/story/index]

In 1969, Dr. Herbert L. Ley, former commissioner of the US Food and Drug Administration [FDA], made a statement that must have shocked even the most vocal critics of the oft-criticized government agency:

The thing that bugs me is that people think the Food and Drug Administration is protecting them-it isn't. What the FDA is doing and what the public thinks it's doing are as different as night and day.

[Source: *In the Name of Science,* Andrew Goliski]

One new drug, the painkiller Vioxx, which was pulled from the market this fall, may have caused 55,000 deaths, a top FDA scientist said recently.

Big Pharma is not beyond scare tactics.

- Big Pharma scare tactics: How the pharmaceutical industry influences American consumers. Sometimes truth is stranger than fiction, especially in this case. Lloyd Grove, a columnist for the New York Daily News, says that the pharmaceutical lobby in the United States, a group called PhRMA, actually commissioned the writing of a fiction novel designed to scare Americans into avoiding prescription drugs from Canada. The book was supposed to tell a story about terrorists who altered prescription drugs from Canada in order to kill Americans who were buying them over the internet or crossing the border to buy them at lower prices. Bizarre, huh? What an interesting tactic to try to convince people to pay sky-high prices-monopoly prices, in fact, for prescription drugs in the United States. But that's only part of this story. When the book project fizzled, the authors were offered $100,000 to keep quiet about the deal, says Grove. The book was also supposed to be "dumbed down" for women, because apparently women make up a large part of the prescription drug buyers in the United States, and the people in charge of this project wanted to make sure women could "understand."

Source: http://healthy.net./scr/news.asp?Id=8432

- Big Pharma markets drugs with the promise to prevent such things as heart attacks, cancer osteoporosis, diabetes and impotence. Unfortunately, many of the drugs being marketed for healthy people to take as a preventative were only tested on sick people. The article in U.S. News & World Report used the example of two drugs called Tambocor and Enkaid. These two drugs were routinely prescribed for years as a preventative of sudden heart attacks. Only after some time did a study of these drugs on healthy people reveal that the drug greatly increased the chance of sudden heart attacks when taken by healthy people. It is estimated that 50,000 people as a result of these drugs may have died before a halt was instituted. The bottom line is that "better living through chemistry" may exact a terrible price.

Source: www.chiropracticresearch.org/NEWSDrugEffects.htm

- In a feature article in the November 16, 1998 issue of the U.S. News & World Report, it was noted that drug usage is actually going up in the US. Drug companies are certainly not crying the blues because of the trend toward health and wellness. In fact they have shifted their emphasis in sales. More and more drug companies are pushing drug usage not only for treatment but for usage before any problems arise as a preventative.[see proceeding paragraph – Big Pharma Markets Drugs]. This mass marketing shift has paid off as prescriptions for drugs went up 400 million from 1993 to 1997, up to an astounding 2.4 billion prescription being dispensed in 1997!

Source: www.chiropracticresearch.org/NEWSDrugEffects.htm.

In my opinion this seems like a left-handed endorsement of the grudging recognition of vitamins and nutritional supplements by Big Pharma. Vitamins and nutritional supplements relegated by them to an underground subculture are starting to rock their vaults. If you don't think so, read about their next strategy by Dr. Carolyn Dean. The pentagon should take lessons from their strategists. Maybe we would have been out of Iraq years ago.

KISS YOUR VITAMINS GOODBYE!

By Dr. Carolyn Dean
June 19, 2005
NewsWithViews.com

The US Delegation to Codex has just issued a formal written statement to the Codex Alimentarius Commission that the United States, during the July 4-9, 2005 meeting in Rome, will support compulsory rules created by this international organization directly overruling US Law regarding access to vitamins.

The US law that is about to be vanquished is the Dietary Supplement, Health and Education Act of 1994. Codex is a joint venture between the United Nation's World

Health Organization. [WHO/FAO] and The World Trade Organization [WTO] who have already stated that it will enforce Codex "guidelines" as the world standard for trade in dietary supplements. This will mean that gradually, pill-by-pill, our access to the dietary supplements we depend on will disappear.

For those not familiar with the Dietary Supplement Health and Education Act of 1994, it was passed because 2.5 million ordinary citizens wanted to make sure dietary supplements such as herbs, vitamins, minerals and other food-based supplements could stay on the over-the-counter market. Movement to create this law, known as DSHEA, started when a 1992 FDA task force published a report announcing the FDA's desire to remove these products from the shelves as they represented a "disincentive for patented drug research".

[Author: I would like to know what members of the 1992 FDA who had sway over the task force that went on a Big Pharma sponsored junket. At the very least they should be fired.]

Immediately following this announcement, millions of Americans learned about how famed vitamin doctor, Jonathan Wright's patient-filled medical office was raided the same month by nearly two-dozen gun-toting, flak-jacketed FDA agents in the name of regulating supplements. Battering down an unlocked office door, these agents, backed by burly sheriff's department deputies, lined up staff and patients against the wall, pulled IV's from patients arms in middle of treatments, confiscated patient records and took the hard drive from the office computer all because Dr. Jonathan Wright was using nutritional supplements to heal very sick people who could not get help from standard allopathic medical care.

As the story developed, it turned out that this Gestapo-style raid was standard operating procedure for the FDA and as the general public became aware of just how many doctors' offices, manufacturing companies, distributors and health food stores had been assaulted by similar raids, the horror of all this forged a mighty health freedom army that resulted in unanimous passage of DSHEA.

The idea of the law was two-fold:

1. DSHEA was to make a clear distinction between FOOD, which is considered generally safe and did not need to have permission from the FDA to be allowed on the market and DRUGS, which are generally toxic, potentially deadly and in need of lengthy evaluation before they were available to the public under prescription from a doctor.

2. DSHEA provides the FDA with plenty of legal authority to remove herbs or dietary supplements from the market providing the agency has plenty of REAL evidence of REAL harm to the public. The FDA also has the authority to limit the amount of a supplement to low levels IF the agency has plenty of REAL evidence to prove higher

levels ARE ACTUALLY dangerous. The FDA will request they be removed from the market.

The FDA and its Big Pharma backers have never liked DSHEA because these products and the related natural healing arts services often related to them are putting the allopathic drug/surgical/chemical medical industry to shame.

In the book, <u>Death by Modern Medicine</u>, using the allopathic medical industry's own official reports, it documents how 784,000 people die every year in the American medical system while following doctors' orders in a highly-regulated allopathic system. The proof that dietary supplements and the practitioners who promote them are safe and work as expected is evidenced everywhere. Studies conducted all over the world have shown that supplements are actually safer than food and there is simply no hard evidence to show there is ANY risk factor worthy of discussion, much less needing universal "risk assessment".

Yet, the US Delegation, along with its Big Pharma backers are bound and determined that Codex force "risk analysis assessments" upon the American dietary supplement industry so they can bypass the expressed will of the American people.

The REAL reason for promotion of "risk assessment" is based on two agendas. First, to be able to strip the over-the-counter marketplace of everything but low quality, low dose-level products that won't do much to support or improve health. Second, to set up the framework to allow Big Pharma to take over the supplement market as a new form of drugs, where prices can be jacked up outrageously and doled out by doctors for a fee.

[Allopathic Medical Care: A system of medical practice that aims to combat disease by use of remedies [as drugs or surgery] producing effects different from or incompatible with those produced by the disease being treated.]

UNDERSTAND THIS: If you do not ACT NOW, you and everyone you love, will be condemned to living under an international law that denies your basic right to maintain your health. WITHOUT HEALTH, YOU HAVE NO FREEDOM!

ACT NOW!   *[Source:* www.friendsoffreedominternational.org]
Related Article:
Codex Alimentaris Ends US Supplements in June 2005.
© 2005 Dr. Carolyn Dean – All Rights Reserved.

Dr. Carolyn Dean is a medical doctor, naturopathic doctor, herbalist, acupuncturist, nutritionist, as well as a powerful health activist fighting for health freedom as president of Friends of Freedom International. Dr. Dean is the author of over a dozen health books, the latest of which is *Death By Modern Medicine.*

Web Site: www.deathbymodernmedicine.com
Source: www.newswithviews.com/guest_opinion/guest60.htm

Note: This chapter or any other chapter in this book is not meant to dispense medical advice or strategies for your health care. It is meant to raise your awareness to be pro-active to other health options which should be discussed with your health care professional.

CHAPTER 7

Vitamins

What are Vitamins?

There are nearly 40 vitamins, minerals, and dietary components that your body needs but cannot manufacture in sufficient amounts. Acting in concert, these essential vitamins and minerals help keep billions of cells healthy and encourage them to grow and reproduce. Some supply the keys to unlocking the energy in the carbohydrate, fat, oils and protein in the foods you eat.

These essentials are often called *micronutrients* because your body needs only tiny amounts of them. Yet failing to get even those small quantities virtually guarantees disease. Old-time sailors learned that living for months without fresh fruits or vegetables—the main sources of vitamin C—causes the bleeding gums and listlessness of scurvy. In some developing countries, people still become blind from vitamin A deficiency. And even in the United States, some children develop the soft, deformed bones of rickets because they don't get enough vitamin D.

Just as a lack of key micronutrients can cause substantial harm to your body, getting sufficient quantities can provide a substantial benefit.

Source: Harvard Medical School.

Before we delve into vitamins, we must first understand the concept of nutrients. To function, the human body must have nutrients. The nutrients known to be essential for human well-being are: proteins, carbohydrates, fats and oils, minerals, vitamins and water.

Vitamins are a group of substances that are essential for normal metabolism – *the process by which substance is handled in the human body* – growth and development, and regulation of cell function. The word 'vitamin' derives from the words vital and amine. Vitamins are organic [that is, carbon containing] molecules which mainly act as a catalyst in our body.

All naturally occurring vitamins are organic food substances that are found only in living things: they are, plants and animals. With a few notable exceptions, the human body cannot manufacture or synthesize vitamins on its own. Vitamins must be supplied in the diet or dietary system, except for vitamin D, which is either synthesized through the skin by the sun's rays or taken as a vitamin.

Vitamins help to regulate the metabolism. Other vitamins also help convert fat and carbohydrates into energy and assist in the formation of healthy bones and tissues. In addition, vitamins provide vitality and general well being.

It is important to understand that vitamins cannot replace food. In fact, vitamins can not be assimilated without ingesting food. **That is why doctors and advocates of natural nutrition stress that vitamins should be taken with meals.** Vitamins work together with enzymes, cofactors and other substances in the digestive tract. As stated earlier, the body can not create vitamin molecules itself. So these molecules must come through food that we eat.

As a general rule, vitamins are destroyed by heat, exposure to air, sunlight, and oxidizing-*to combine with oxygen by exposure to air-* conditions. Improper storage conditions can allow mold growth. If mixed into other foods, vitamins should always be consumed within a couple of days at most.

Researchers have found that the requirement of vitamins varies from one person to another, and that psychological stress can rapidly delete the body's vitamin reserves. Within a few notable exceptions, such as vitamin A, D, B6, and potassium, it is better to have an excess of vitamins·in the body than to be deficient. Vitamin supplements are readily available at health food stores, pharmacies and grocery stores, and are usually inexpensive.

Each vitamin plays a specific role in the human body. In many cases, vitamins must interact with other vitamins to function properly, and a lack of any one of them can disturb the assimilation of another vitamin. Thus, taking multi-vitamin formulas where there is too much of one vitamin and too little of another can have less then desirable results. **Poorly balanced multi-vitamin formulas can even cause vitamin deficiencies.**

Please bear in mind that vitamins are not toxic, although an overdose of certain vitamins can have adverse effects, such as Vitamin A [retinal, retinal and retinoic acid] and Vitamin D. *To avoid overdosing Vitamin A, take a low dose of Beta Carotene and the body will convert the proper amount of Vitamin A it requires.*

Wading through Alphabet Soup. *Source:* Harvard Medical School.

In 1941, the U.S. Food and Nutrition Board published the first in a series of reports on recommended dietary allowances [RDAs]. These reports set forth the amounts of various nutrients needed to avoid deficiency diseases. Six decades and hundreds of studies later, another panel of scientists released the dietary reference intakes [DRI's]. These evidence-based standards go beyond amending deficiencies, they also suggest the amounts of nutrients needed to enhance health in many ways.

To show people how much of each micronutrient they should get, the DRI lists either the familiar RDA or another measure called *adequate intake* [AI], plus additional information. The explanations below will help you wade through this maze of acronyms.

 ▪ **Recommended dietary allowance [RDA].** This is the average daily amount of a nutrient necessary to meet the requirements of almost all [97%-98%] healthy people in a specific life stage category. The factors that distinguish life stage categories are age, sex, pregnancy, and nursing.

 ▪ **Adequate intake [AI].** *Adequate intake* is an estimate used when there are not enough data to support an RDA. This figure is the amount of a nutrient that's believed to be adequate for healthy people. Again, recommendations may differ depending on life stage.

- **Tolerable upper intake [UL].** The *tolerable upper intake level* is the highest amount of a nutrient deemed likely to have no harmful effects on almost all healthy people when taken consistently. When people take more than the UL, the risk of side effects rises with the dose.

- **Estimated average requirement [EAR].** The *estimated average requirement* is the daily amount of a nutrient estimated to fulfill the needs of half the healthy people in a specific group. This level would not meet the needs of the other half of the group. EAR's aren't useful to the general public; scientific panels use them to help determine RDA's and AI's.

To help people apply these vitamin and mineral guidelines to their daily food choices, the FDA created the "Nutrition Facts" panel that appears on almost all packaged foods. Nearly every can, bag, or box you toss into your shopping cart will have a printed description of what's inside. This includes the percentages of *daily values [DV's] of each nutrient in a single serving of the food, as well as other important information such as serving size, calories preserving, and amounts of fat, sodium, carbohydrate and protein.*

Daily values don't take life stage categories into account. They're based on the highest daily allowance value and are presented as percentages calculated for a person eating 2,000-2,5000 calories a day—a diet that supplies more energy than many inactive people need for maintaining a healthy weight.

According to your doctor the best way to ensure that your body gets the daily requirement of vitamins is to eat a balanced diet, which contains a variety of foods. The daily recommended levels of vitamins are often referred to as the RDA or Recommended Daily Allowances.

Today we have the RDA put forward by the Food and Nutritional Board of the National Research Counsel. The RDA's are the minimum requirement of nutrition: you can barely survive on them. The RDA for vitamin C will keep you from getting scurvy, but doesn't protect you well from the onslaught of environmental toxins.

Vitamins can be used to effectively treat and cure nutritional based deficiencies. Although vitamins do not prevent or cure other types of invasive diseases such as cancer, afflictions related to aging or biological infections, a diet that supplies the proper balance of essential vitamins and nutrients can help fortify the immune system and thus provide some beneficial protection against such diseases. It is likely that future discoveries will shed new light on vitamins and their important role in human disease.

Source: http://vu.org/staffl/example2.html

There are many nutritionists that would like to see the RDA replaced with the ODA, or Optimum Daily Allowances which would be based upon an individuals age, lifestyle and locations [since the quality of our air and water changes from location to location].

Scurvy is probably the first illness [which was later recognized] as a nutritional deficiency disorder. Hippocrates first described scurvy, in the fifth century, as bleeding gums, hemorrhaging, and death. However it wasn't until 1747, when the Scottish physician James Lind aboard the Salisbury experimented with a number of food combinations on patients suffering from scurvy that the British Admiralty started to pay attention. Lind discovered that those who were given an orange and lemon combination recovered, and recovered quite swiftly. When the colonies revolted, the Colonial Army too used fruit to keep their soldiers healthy, while some were treated to the Native American infusion of pine bark and needles when fruit was out of season, "In 1795," Dr. Anderson tells us, "the Admiralty finally mandated lemon juice for all sailors." [A Short History of Scurvy, Mark R. Anderson, MD 2000]

According to Albert Szent-Gyrogyi the Noble-prize winner for his discovery of vitamin C, "The medical profession itself took a very narrow and very wrong view. Lack of ascorbic acid caused scurvy so if there was no scurvy there was no lack of ascorbic acid. Nothing could be clearer than this, the only trouble was that scurvy is not a first symptom, it's after the fact, of a lack but final collapse, a premortal syndrome and there is a very wide gap between scurvy and full health."

1860 Louis Pasteur discovered that microscopic organisms caused man diseases. His discovery prompted further research into the curative and preventative properties of vitamins.

1906 English biochemist Sir Fredrick G. Hopkins discovered certain food factors were important to health. Christian Eijkman and Hopkins shared the 1929 Noble prize in medicine, but Eijkman's greatest contribution to medicine was discovering how wrong one can be while blindly sticking to one's guns: he learned to allow the scientific process to determine truth. Sir Hopkins had established the methodology in an experiment whereby he fed mice "a synthetic diet of pure carbohydrate, pure protein, fats, and salts, Hopkins observed that the mice would stop growing unless their diet was supplemented with milk. The milk, he concluded, must contain small amounts of what he called "additional food factors" in order for growth and the maintenance of health. Hopkins succeeded in isolation it became known as vitamins A and D." [Hopkins, Sir Fredrick Gowland. "Microsoft Encarta Encyclopedia"].

Thus by depriving animals of different types of foods in controlled experiments, scientists could now identify a number of different substances that would be soon classified as "vitamins". Here we have both the beginning of the nutritional sciences and the initial roots and the reason for the formation of the organization, People for the Ethical Treatment of Animals [PETA].

Pellagra is a disease that was common throughout the world in the 19th century, and still exists in some parts of the world.. It has been a little too common in the poor south, and with the economic downturn and crop failure of the early 1900's, pellagra had blossomed into a full blown epidemic. The disease caused skin rashes, especially when exposed to sunlight, mouth lesions, diarrhea, and if left long enough, mental deterioration. In 1914 the surgeon general appointed Dr. Joseph Goldberger, a member of the public health service for fifteen years, to tackle the crisis of pellagra. Goldberger first merely observed the disease. He took notes, asked questions, and watched. He noted that the diet of the poor in the region consisted of cornbread, molasses and some pork fat. The poorer the people the more likely they were to get pellagra. He noted that the institutions, prisons, orphanages and asylums had many cases of pellagra.

At the time, the germ theory of disease had taken hold of medical thought, and it was assumed that pellagra was an infectious disease. Additionally, society is hardly ever ready to accept the idea that poverty could possibly cause a disease. So when Goldberger concluded that pellagra was a nutritional disease, the medical community was less than happy to receive this news.

So in order to prove his theory, Dr. Goldberger approached a prison to ask their aid in conducting a nutritional study. The prisoners who volunteered for the experiment would be pardoned. He did his best to separate the two groups so that infectious disease could be ruled out. Because it was a farm prison and their basic nutrition was good, there were no cases of pellagra. Goldberger separated his two groups, gave his experimental group the diet of the southern poor: cornmeal, molasses, and pork fat, and sure enough, within a few months, his experimental group came down with pellagra. Then to test whether pellagra was infectious, the researchers tried to "catch" the disease from the ill prisoners, but were unable. Finally, when given meat, fresh vegetables, and mild, the pellagra symptoms vanished.

Still, given this evidence, the medical community was unwilling to accept his study. Goldberger tried repeatedly to convince others but eventually gave up and spent the rest of his life looking for the "exact" *nutritional factor that caused pellagra*, but it would be discovered only after his death. Goldberger's career carried him to Washington DC where he had researched infectious diseases for an organization that would eventually become the National Institute of Health.

1911 Polish scientist Casmir Funk named special nutritional parts of food as "vitamine" after "vita" meaning life and amine from a compound in thiamine he isolated in rice husks. Vitamine was later shortened to vitamin. *Together Hopkins and Funk formed the Vitamin Hypothesis of Deficiency disease, stating that lack of vitamins could make you ill. From the initial discovery of vitamins in 1911 through the 1950's nearly all the physicians around the world based their studies and diagnoses on vitamin deficiencies.* During the 1940's and 1950's a number of researchers began to lay the foundation for a new era in vitamins. Much of our present day knowledge evolved from the work of other scientists.

1922 Vitamin E discovered by University of California researchers Herbert Evans and Katherine Bishop
1922 Vitamin D discovered by Edward Mellanby while researching rickets.
1926 B-2 discovered by DTS Smith and EG Hendricks.
1930 many more discoveries were made in the world of biochemical nutrition and all the vitamins were named.
1931 Albert Szent-Györgyi and a fellow researcher Joseph Svirely determined that "hexuronic acid" was actually vitamin C and noted its anti-scorbutic activity. In 1937, Szent-Györgyi was awarded the Noble Prize for his discovery. In 1943 Edward Adelbert Doisy and Henrik Dara were awarded the Nobel Prize for their discovery of vitamin K and its chemical structure.

1933 Folic acid discovered by Lucy Weller.
1934 B-6 discovered by Paul Gyorgy.
1937 Niacin discovered by Conrad Elvehjem and as well as discovering that the B vitamins, nicotinic acid or niacin prevented and cured pellagra.

Vitamins are classified as either water-soluble, meaning that they dissolve easily in water, or fat-soluble, and are absorbed through the intestinal tract with the help of lipids. Each vitamin is typically used in multiple reactions and, therefore, most have multiple functions.

Vitamin Name	Chemical Name	Solubility	Diseases Caused by Deficiency	Recommended Dietary Allowances [male, age 19-70]	Upper Intake Level [UL/day]
Vitamin A	Retinoids [restinol, retinoids and carotenoids]	Fat	Night-blindness Keratoinalacis	900 mg	3,000 mg
Vitamin B_1	Thiamine	Water	Beriberi	1.2 mg	[N/D]
Vitamin B_2	Riboflavin	Water	Ariboflavinosis	1.3 mg	N/D
Vitamin B_3	Niacin	Water	Pellagra	16.0 mg	35.0 mg
Vitamin B_3	Pantothenic acid	Water	Paresthesia	5.0 mg	N/D
Vitamin B_6	Pyridoxine	Water	Anemia	1.3-1.7 mg	100 mg
Vitamin B_7	Biotin	Water	None Identified	30.0 mg	N/D
Vitamin B_9	Folic Acid	Water	May be linked to heart disease & cancer. Deficiency during pregnancy is associated with birth defects such as neural tube defects.	400 mg	1,000 mg
Vitamin B_{12}	Cyanocobala-min	Water	Megaloblastio anaemia	2.4 mg	N/D
Vitamin C	Ascorbic Acid	Water	Scurvy	90.0 mg	2,000 mg
Vitamin D*	Ergocalciferol Cholecalci-ferol	Fat	Rickets, Osteomalacia	5.0 mg-10 mg	50 mg
Vitamin E	Tocopherol, Tocotrienol	Fat	Deficiency is very rare, mild hemolytic anemia in newborn infants.	15.0 mg	1,000 mg
Vitamin K	Naphtho-quinene	Fat	Bleeding diathesis	120 mg	N/D

*Vitamin D is the only vitamin your body manufactures through the process of your skin to exposure of the sun.

A prescribed dietary supplement is intended to supply nutrients [vitamins, minerals, fatty acids or amino acids] that are missing or not consumed in sufficient quantity in a person's diet. This may include herbal supplements which have a history of claims that they cure or prevent certain diseases. The medical utility and regulation status of dietary supplements is controversial.

In the United States, a dietary supplement is defined under the Dietary Supplement Health and Education Act of 1994 as a product that meets each of the following criteria:

1. It is intended to supplement the <u>diet</u> and bears or contains one or more of the following dietary ingredients:
>   a <u>vitamin,</u>
>   a <u>mineral,</u>
>   an <u>herb</u> or other <u>botanical</u> [excluding tobacco],
>   an <u>amino acid,</u>
>   a dietary substance for use by man to supplement the diet by increasing the total daily intake [e.g., <u>enzymes,</u> or <u>tissues</u> from <u>organs</u> or <u>glands</u>],
>   a concentrate, such as a meal replacement or <u>energy bar,</u> or
>   a metabolite, constituent, or extract.

2. It is intended for ingestion in pill, capsule, tablet, or liquid form.

3. It is not represented for use as a conventional food or as the sole item of a meal or diet.

4. It is labeled as a "dietary supplement".

The <u>FDA</u> regulates dietary supplements as foods, and not as <u>drugs.</u> The FDA does not pre-approve dietary supplements on their safety and efficacy, unlike drugs. In contrast, the FDA can only go after dietary supplement manufacturers after they have put unsafe products on the market. However, certain foods [such as <u>infant formula</u> and medical foods] are deemed special nutritionals because they are consumed by highly vulnerable populations and are thus regulated more strictly than the majority of dietary supplements.

The claims that a dietary supplement makes are essential to its classification. If a dietary supplement claims in any way to cure, mitigate, or treat a disease, it would be considered to be an unauthorized new drug and in violation of the applicable regulations and statutes. As the FDA states it in a response to this question in <u>FAQ</u>:

Is it legal to market a dietary supplement product as a treatment or cure for a specific disease or condition?

No, a product sold as a dietary supplement and promoted on its label or in labeling* as a treatment, prevention or cure for a specific disease or condition would be considered an unapproved –and thus illegal – drug. To maintain the product's status as a dietary supplement, the label, and labeling must be consistent with the provisions in the Dietary Supplement Health and Education Act. [DSHEA] of 1994.

Labeling refers to the label as well as accompanying material that is used by a manufacturer to promote and market a specific product.

Vitamin deficiencies

Deficiencies of vitamins are classified as either primary or secondary. A primary deficiency occurs when you do not get enough of the vitamin in the food you eat. A secondary deficiency may be due to an underlying disorder that prevents or limits the absorption or use of the vitamin, due to a "lifestyle factor", such as smoking, excessive alcohol consumption, or the use of medications that interfere with the absorption or the body's use of the vitamin. Individuals who eat a varied diet are unlikely to develop a severe primary vitamin deficiency. In contrast, restrictive diets have the potential to cause prolonged vitamin deficits, which may result in often painful and potentially deadly diseases.

Because humans do not store most vitamins in their bodies, a human must consume them regularly to avoid deficiency. Vitamins A, D, and B are stored in significant amounts in the human body, mainly in the liver, and an adult human may be deficient in Vitamin A and B for long periods of time before developing a deficiency condition. Vitamin B is not stored in the human body in significant amounts, so it may only last a couple of days.

Well-known human vitamin deficiencies involve thiamine [beriberi], niacin [pellagra], vitamin C [scurvy] and vitamin D [rickets]. In much of the developed world, such deficiencies are rare; this is due to an adequate supply of food; and the addition of vitamins and minerals, often called fortification, to common foods.

Vitamin Side Effects and Overdose

In large doses some vitamins have documented side effects. Vitamin side effects tend to increase in severity with increasing dosage. The likelihood of consuming too much of any vitamin from food is remote, but overdosing from vitamin supplementation does occur. At high enough dosages some vitamins cause side effects, such as nausea, diarrhea, and vomiting. Unlike some of the side effects caused by drugs, vitamin side effects rarely cause any permanent harm. When vitamin side effects emerge, recovery is often accomplished by reducing the dosage. Furthermore, the concentrations of vitamins an individual can tolerate vary widely and appear to be related to age and state of health.

Approximately 150 million people use supplements each year, but just 240 deaths have been attributed to supplements from 1994 to 2004 [the most recent years for which we have statistics]. That averages out to about 22 supplement-related deaths each year. *Comparing this with 305,000 deaths per year due to adverse drug reactions, it is inconceivable that traditional medicine is not more open to the use of nutritional supplements.* What's more, most of those deaths were linked to products that contained ephedra [which was subsequently banned by the FDA]. And the problem wasn't actually the ephedra itself – it was the use of ephedra products in combination with caffeine, a practice that the product's label warned against. The result was a risky recipe that could, and did, cause deadly ventricular fibrillation.

Source: *Heart, Health & Nutrition*, March 2007.

There is a caveat [warning] I have come upon in my research regarding a commonly known nutrient:

- Selenium. It seems a recent study of over 9,000 U.S. residents found diabetes was more common among those with high blood selenium levels. It seems advisable to keep your selenium in normal ranges.

  Sources: J. Am. Med. Assoc. 276: 1957, 1998; *J. Natl. Cancer Inst.*95:1477, 2003; *Ann. Intern. Med.* 147:217, 2007; *Diabetes Care* 30: 829, 2007; *J. Am. Coll. Nutr.* 24:250, 2005.

Before we leave the chapter on Vitamins, these are some of the statements you may have heard and were afraid to ask about.

What does "bioavailability" mean? Bio means *life* or *living system*, and ***available*** means *ready for use*. So, bioavailability is the degree and rate at which a substance is absorbed into a living system or is made available to the body.

What are "oxidation reactions"? Oxidation reactions occur when a substance combines with oxygen. Oxidation reactions are necessary for body functions. These reactions can cause damage if the oxygen becomes "reactive" by becoming peroxide or a single oxygen.

What is "oxidative stress"? Oxidative stress describes a process in which there is an increase in free radicals that damages cells and causes disease. When this happens, the body does not maintain its healthy antioxidant protection and hosts free radicals.

What are free radicals? Free radicals are aggressive chemicals that cause permanent damage when they react with cell components. They are atoms or molecules that have an unpaired electron that makes them highly reactive. Free radicals attack the nearest stable molecule and "steal" its electron. When a stable molecule is attached it becomes a free radical itself, creating a chain that can eventually cause cell damage. There has been an association between free radicals and premature aging and the development of degenerative diseases.

What are antioxidants? Antioxidant is a catchall term for any compound that can counteract unstable molecules that damage DNA, cell membranes, and other parts of cells. These unstable molecules may be *free radicals*, oxygen free radicals, reactive oxygen species, or reactive nitrogen species. Free radicals are a natural by-product of energy metabolism and are also generated by ultraviolet rays, tobacco smoke, and air pollution. They lack a full complement of electrons, which makes them unstable, so they steal electrons from other molecules, damaging those molecules in the process. One example of this harm is when free radicals attack low-density lipoproteins [LDL, the "bad" cholesterol] that have made their way into the cells lining artery walls. After giving up the electrons, the LDL molecules become more reactive compounds that can injure the arterial lining and spark a cascade of events that can eventually narrow the artery if repeated over time.

Antioxidants are able to neutralize marauders such as free radicals by giving up some of their own electrons. When a vitamin C or E molecule makes this sacrifice, it may allow a crucial protein gene or cell membrane to escape damage. This helps break a chain reaction that can affect many other cells.

Your body cells naturally produce plenty of antioxidants to put on patrol. The foods you eat—and perhaps some of the supplements you take—are another source of antioxidant compounds. *Carotenoids* [such as lycopene in tomatoes and lutein in kale] and *flavonoids* [such as anthocyanins in blueberries, quercetin in apples and onions, and catechins in green tea act as antioxidants. So do vitamins C and E, *beta carotene*, and the mineral selenium, which are among the most studied antioxidants.

Source: Harvard Medical School, "Understanding Antioxidants."

What is beta carotene? A precursor that is converted by the body into vitamin A. Beta carotene acts as an antioxidant. It's found in many green vegetables and dark yellow or deep orange fruits and vegetables. I recommend only taking beta carotene for your vitamin A needs. The body converts beta carotene to the vitamin as your body requires.

What is bone mineral density? The amount of mineralized bone tissue in a given area; usually calculated in grams per square centimeter.

What are carotenoids? Plant and animal pigments that color many fruits and vegetables, including carrots and cantaloupe. Some carotenoids can be converted to vitamin A.

What are dietary supplements? Vitamins, minerals, herbs, amino acids, enzymes, organ tissues, and a few other substances promoted as a way to bolster diet, Unlike drugs, they are not regulated by the FDA.

What are flavonoids? An antioxidant substance found in tea, berries, tomatoes, and onions, among other sources.

What is hemochromatosis? An excess of iron that may damage body tissues and raise risks for infection, heart disease, liver, cancer, and arthritis. Causes include a genetic glitch, large doses of ion supplements, multiple blood transfusions, alcoholism, and some rare metabolic disorders.

What is homocysteine? A protein by-product that appears to increase the risk of heart disease and strokes when present in the blood at high levels.

What are micronutrients? Nutrients such as vitamins and minerals that the body requires in fairly small quantities.

What are oxalates? Substances in fiber, roots, rhubarb, and spinach that bind with calcium so the body cannot absorb it.

What are phytates? Substances in whole grain, legumes, and seeds that bind with certain micronutrients, such as iron, calcium, magnesium, copper, and zinc, so that they pass through the intestines instead of being absorbed and used by the body.

What are phytochemicals? Compounds in plants that affect their taste, color, scent, and other properties. Lycopene, found in tomatoes, is one phytochemical thought to have beneficial effects for humans.

What is a precursor? A substance that the body can convert into the active form of a vitamin. One example is beta carotene, which the body can convert into vitamin A as needed.

What are Minerals?

Vitamins alone are not enough.
Source: Earl Mendell's Vitamin Bible

As important as vitamins are, they can do nothing for you without minerals. I like to call minerals the Cinderellas of the nutrition world, because, though very few people are aware of it, vitamins cannot function, cannot be assimilated, without the aid of minerals. And though the body can synthesize some vitamins, it cannot manufacture a *single* mineral.

Major Minerals   *Source:* Harvard Medical School

The body needs, and stores, fairly large amounts of the major minerals, as shown below.
- Calcium
- Chloride
- Magnesium
- Phosphorus
- Potassium
- Sodium
- Sulfur

These minerals are no more important to your health than the trace minerals; they're just present in your body in greater amounts. One of their key tasks is maintaining the proper balance of water in the body. Sodium chloride, and potassium take the lead in doing this. Three other major minerals—calcium, phosphorus, and magnesium—are important for healthy bones. Sulfur helps stabilize protein structures, including some of those that make up hair, skin, and nails.

Major minerals travel through the body in various ways. Potassium, for example, is quickly absorbed into the bloodstream, where it circulates freely and is excreted by the kidneys, much like a water-soluble vitamin. Calcium is more like a fat-soluble vitamin because it requires vitamin D as a carrier for absorption and transport.

Having too much of one major mineral can result in a deficiency of another. Calcium binds with excess sodium in the body and is excreted when the body senses that sodium levels must be lowered. That means that if you get too much sodium through table salt or processed foods, you could end up losing needed calcium as your body rids itself of the surplus sodium. Likewise, too much phosphorous can hamper your ability to absorb magnesium. Often, these sorts of imbalances are caused by overloads from supplements, not food sources.

Trace Minerals   *Source:* Harvard Medical School

A thimble could easily contain the distillation of all the trace minerals normally found in your body [see below]:

- Chromium
- Copper
- Fluoride
- Iodine
- Iron
- Manganese
- Selenium
- Zinc

Yet their contributions are just as essential as those of major minerals such as calcium and phosphorous, which each account for more than a pound of your body weight. Trace minerals carry out a diverse set of tasks. Iron, for example, is best known for ferrying oxygen throughout the body, while fluoride strengthens bones and wards off tooth decay. Zinc helps blood clot, is essential for taste and smell, and bolsters the immune response. Copper helps form several enzymes, one of which assists with iron metabolism and the creation of hemoglobin, which carries oxygen in the blood. The other trace minerals perform equally vital jobs, such as helping to block damage to body cells and forming parts of key enzymes or enhancing their activity.

Trace minerals interact with one another, sometimes in ways that can trigger imbalances. Too much of one can cause or contribute to a deficiency of another; for example, a minor overload of manganese can exacerbate iron deficiency. Having too little can also cause problems. When the body has too little iodine, thyroid hormone production slows, causing sluggishness and weight gain as well as other health concerns. The problem worsens if the body also has too little selenium. The difference between "just enough" and "too much" of the trace minerals is often tiny. Generally, food is a safe source of trace minerals, but if you take supplements, it's important to make sure you're not exceeding safe levels.

What are Water- and Fat-soluble Vitamins?
Source: Harvard Medical School

Water-soluble Vitamins [*Water-soluble vitamins are usually depleted in the body in approximately 48 hours, with exceptions of vitamin B-12 which can be stored in the body for longer periods.*]

Although water-soluble vitamins [see below] have many tasks in the body, one of the most important is helping to free the energy found in the food you eat. Vitamin B-12 is bound to protein in food. Hydrochloric acid in the stomach releases B-12 from the protein during digestion. As we get into our 40s and 50s, there is a depletion of hydrochloric acid available for digestion causing deficiency of B-12. It is therefore prudent to take a B-12 sublingual supplement [used under the tongue] to make up the deficiency.

B vitamins:
- Biotin
- Folic acid [folate]
- Niacin [Vitamin B]
- Pantothenic acid
- Riboflavin [vitamin B]
- Thiamin [vitamin B] B1
- Vitamin B_6 [pyridoxine]
- Vitamin B_{12} [cyanocobalamin]
- Vitamin C

Several B vitamins are key components of certain coenzymes [molecules that aid enzymes] that help release that energy. Thiamin, riboflavin, niacin, pantothenic acid, and biotin engage in energy production. Vitamins B_6 and B_{12}, and folic acid metabolize amino acids [the building blocks of proteins] and help cells multiply. One of many roles played by vitamin C is to help make collagen, which knits together wounds, supports blood vessel walls, and forms a base for teeth and bones.

Water-soluble vitamins are packed into the watery portions of the foods you eat. They are absorbed directly into the bloodstream as food is broken down during digestion or as a supplement dissolves. Because much of your body consists of water, many of the water-soluble vitamins circulate easily in your body.

Contrary to popular belief, water-soluble vitamins can stay in the body for short [approx. 24 to 48 hours] periods of time. Generally, though, water-soluble vitamins should be replenished every one to three days.

There is a small risk that consuming very large amounts of some of these micronutrients through supplements may be quite harmful. Very high doses of B_6, for example, can damage nerves, causing numbness and muscle weakness. High doses of potassium can adversely affect your heart rhythm.

Fat-soluble Vitamins [*Fat-soluble vitamins are usually depleted in the body in approx. 10 days.*]

Bone formation would be stymied without vitamins A, D, and K, three of the four fat-soluble vitamins listed below:
- Vitamin A
- Vitamin D
- Vitamin E
- Vitamin K

Vitamin A also helps keep cells healthy and protects your vision. Without vitamin E, the remaining fat-soluble vitamin, your body would have difficulty absorbing and storing vitamin A. Vitamin E also acts as an *antioxidant* [a compound that helps protect the body against damage from unstable molecules]. Together, the quartet helps keep your eyes, skin, lungs, gastrointestinal tract, and nervous system in good repair.

Rather than slipping into the bloodstream like most water-soluble vitamins, fat-soluble vitamins gain entry to the blood via lymph channels in the intestinal walls. Many fat-soluble vitamins travel through the body only under escort by proteins that act as carriers. Fatty foods and oils are reservoirs for the fat-soluble vitamins. Within your body, fat tissues and the liver act as the main holding pens for these vitamins and release them as needed. To some extent, you can think of these vitamins as time-release micronutrients. It's possible to consume them every now and again, perhaps in doses weeks and months apart rather than daily, and still get your fill. Your body squirrels away the excess and doles it out gradually to meet your needs. Because these vitamins are stored for long periods, however, toxic levels can build up. This is most likely to happen if you take supplements beyond recommended dosage of a health care provider. It's very rare to get too much of a vitamin just from food.

Vitamins
All Nutritional Supplements are Not Created Equal.

The FDA regulates dietary supplements as foods, and not as <u>drugs</u>. The FDA does not pre-approve dietary supplements on their safety and efficacy, unlike drugs. In contrast, the FDA can only go after dietary supplement manufacturers after they have put unsafe products on the market.

Let the buyer beware:
All Nutritional Supplements are not created equal.

The FDA classifies supplements into three broad categories.

- Animal grade
  obviously not for you and me, but our pets.
- Food grade
  I qualify this as the lowest grade. You should avoid and <u>not buy</u>.
- USP Pharmaceutical grade
  My research indicates there is no protocol for USD pharmaceutical grade. That is to say this term is a misnomer and is very misleading, allowing the buying public to believe that the product is as reliable as a supposedly well-tested prescription drug.
  This obviously has the pharmaceutical industry's tentacles around it. You usually need a doctor's prescription for it. You will usually pay a higher price for it and it is not necessary.
- *The FDA does not list [GMP]as a category as it is not controlled by the pharmaceutical industry, which was set up by the National Nutritional Food Association [NNFA].*

The NNFA is a governing association certifying the Good Manufacturing Practices [GMP]. It is your assurance that you are receiving the purest ingredients in the proper concentrations.

Program Objectives

The NNFA [Natural Products Association] GMP Certification Program is designed to verify compliance of member suppliers of dietary supplements with a standardized set of good manufacturing practices [GMPs] developed by NNFA. This program is based upon third party inspections of member suppliers and comprehensive audits of their GMP programs in the areas of Personnel, Plant and Grounds, Sanitation, Equipment, Quality Operations, Production and Process Controls, Warehouse, Distribution and Post-Distribution Practices. This program ensures that all elements of the manufacturing process are reviewed to provide reasonable assurance that processes are sufficiently controlled so that products meet their purported quality.

Member suppliers that meet minimum NNFA GMPs standards and have received an "A" compliance rating after an NNFA GMP audit will be entitled to apply for certification and use of the NNFA GMP certification mark. NNFA certification and display of the GMP certification mark demonstrate to retailers, consumers and the public-at-large that products have been manufactured using good manufacturing practices and bring a means of self-assurance to the dietary supplement industry.

Organization – NNFA

The NNFA, the largest dietary supplement trade association in the United States, has developed GMP standards based upon dialogs with member suppliers, other trade associations, and the FDA. The NNFA GMPs are a living document and will be updated periodically based upon feedback from consultants, member companies, best quality practices and the FDA, NNFA will facilitate certification of member suppliers by providing education and training upon request

GMP Advisory Committee

The GMP Advisory Committee, under the direct supervision of NNFA, is comprised of three experts selected for their expertise and training in GMPs. Whenever possible, the Committee members will have a diverse background, including food, dietary supplements, pharmaceuticals, and botanicals, representing the needs of membership.

The functions of the Advisory Committee include:
- Periodic review of the NNFA GMPs
- Review and revision of suggested programs, procedures and records, necessary to meet GMPs
- Review and revision of the Audit Checklist and Performance Rating System
- Selection of auditing companies and assessment of their performance.
- Resolution of any disagreements between auditors and member suppliers.

Audits will be conducted by experienced auditors that have been trained in the NNFA GMPs and performance rating system, and have the required education, experience and training to conduct on-site audits. Typical education and experience of auditors is:
- A four year college degree in biology, chemistry, or food sciences.
- Expertise in food or pharmaceutical GMPs

- Experience in the manufacturing processes for foods or dietary supplements
- Successful completion of training in the NNFA GMPs

Auditors are responsible for all phases of the audits, including completion of the audit checklist, the audit report follow-up on corrective actions, and any secondary audits.

Performance Rating System

The levels of compliance are as follows:

A. A member supplier has excellent compliance with NNFA GMPs, with few deficiencies noted.

B. A member supplier has good compliance with NNFA GMPs, but several significant deficiencies were noted.

C. A member supplier has fair or poor compliance with NNFA GMPs, many deficiencies noted; a re-audit of the facility required.

The compliance ratings determine need for corrective actions and follow-up inspections.

Member suppliers earning an "A" rating may immediately apply to NNFA for certification and the right to use the NNFA Certification mark. Member suppliers earning a "B" rating may apply to NNFA for re-certification and use of the certification mark once there is written verification that the outstanding deficiencies have been corrected. Member suppliers earning a "C" rating may apply to the NNFA for re-certification and use of the certification mark after successful completion of a second audit and once there is written verification that outstanding deficiencies have been corrected.

Certification Procedure

Once a member company has documented compliance with NNFA GMPs, they may apply to NNFA for certification and the right to use the GMP certification mark. The application will be reviewed together with the audit and corrective action reports. Upon successful completion of certification, the official NNFA GMP certification mark may be used on the member supplier's labels, marketing and advertisements. Certification will be valid for a period of no more than three years from the date of the award.

As you can see, the GMP label is given only to supplements manufacturers who meet these strict standards. I would not buy any supplement without that label.

In my experience and with all the research I have done, the majority – *with a very small exception* – of multi-vitamin formulas on the market today give the user a false sense of security – *because of inadequate formulas which usually follow the government's recommended daily allowance [RDAs] which based on available scientific literature are absurdly low* – that they are getting the adequate amounts on the label of the nutrients that are listed.

My Vitamins

What's doing with your body nutrition-wise after taking all of those nutritional supplements you're talking about?

It's funny you should ask.

Over the last 45 years I had researched all of the supplements I was taking to prevent the risks factors of deficiency diseases they were recommended to prevent.

Dosages and additional supplements were adjusted up or down. Supplements were added or deleted. Dosages were adjusted up or down according to changing research and also by two alternative/integrated cardiologists I had been seeing.

I was never sick, but always wondered whether I should take less supplements or more supplements, and are the dosages optimal.

The lab work I had, indicated normal serum levels of folic acid, B-12, Vit D, calcium and potassium. These tests never gave functional levels, which would indicate:
- What the correct dosage levels should be
- How effective is a particular supplement I am taking?
- Should I be eliminating some supplements because they are not necessary?
- Should I add a supplement I am not taking, which is necessary?

The functioning evaluations were introduced to me by Dr. Scott Banks, Doctor of Chiropractic and Nutritional Counseling of Huntington, New York.

He introduced me to Functional Intracellular Analysis [FIA] available exclusively through a patented process of Spectracel Laboratories.

This process measures levels of selected vitamins, minerals and other essential micronutrients within your white blood cells [lymphocytes].

If you decided to fine-tune the supplements you are taking, these tests are not covered by most insurance companies, including Medicare.

The future of nutritional medicine holds wondrous possibilities for mankind, and as our knowledge of vitamins and other nutrients expands further, we will no doubt discover that vitamins have even greater value and utility then we presently imagine.

Source: http://www.mdwelldir.org/docs/history/vitamin.html

Note: This chapter or any other chapter in this book is not meant to dispense medical advice or strategies for your health care. It is meant to raise your awareness to be pro-active to other health options which should be discussed with your health care professional.

CHAPTER 8

What Are Antioxidants and Free Radicals?

An antioxidant can be a vitamin, phytochemical, or mineral. Antioxidants neutralize damage to the body's cells and are naturally present in vegetables, fruits, whole grains, beans and nuts.

Research studies have found growing evidence that antioxidants may protect the body's cells from the kind of cell damage that can lead to cancer.

Over the past two decades, scientists have studied antioxidants like vitamins C and E. Other antioxidants being investigated are phytochemicals like beta-carotene [related to vitamin A], lycopene, lutein and reservatrol, as well as the trace mineral selenium.

Foods that have high amounts of antioxidants are often easy to identify, because many are bright colored. For example, carrots and sweet potatoes have plenty of beta-carotene; bell peppers, strawberries and tomatoes contain vitamin C; tomatoes and watermelon have lycopene; and dark leafy greens like spinach contain lutein. Broccoli has plenty of beta-carotene and vitamin C among its many protective compounds. Blueberries have anthocyanins. Red grapes have reservatrol. Many herbs – including oregano, rosemary and parsley contain a range of antioxidants.

Why Do Our Bodies Need Antioxidants?

Antioxidants defend the body's cells against molecules called "free radicals."

It's one of life's great ironies: The same oxygen we need to live can also do serious harm over time. Cellular activities that keep us alive also produce destructive oxygen molecules in the highly reactive, unstable form of free radicals.

Free radicals possess an unpaired electron. Pairing this lone electron with another gives the molecule stability. To achieve stability, a free radical scavenges electrons from other molecules, which disrupts their stability in turn. This process can start a chemical chain reaction that produces even more free radicals.

In addition to the free radicals produced by normal body processes as we age, our cells must also contend with free radicals that result from such common hazards as ultra-violet light, x-rays, heat, cigarette smoke, alcohol and some pollutants.

Free radicals can do some good, as well. They have the ability to destroy potentially harmful cells, such as bacteria, that invade the body. But too many free radicals can inflict damage to healthy cells. Research now implicates excess free radicals in a number of diseases, including cancer.

For example, a damaged cell may not activate its natural cancer-fighting defenses. It also may fail in some of its other chemical functions, or even pass on damaged DNA as it divides into new cells. If uncorrected, damage can accumulate and result in disease.

How Do Antioxidants Work?

Fortunately, antioxidants in our diet can help offset damage caused by free radicals.

Dietary antioxidants function in a variety of ways. They can limit free radical formation, destroy free radicals, stimulate antioxidant enzyme activity and stimulate enzymes' repair activity.

Many scientists believe that a plentiful supply of antioxidants, carrying out different protective roles, may help defend against the cell changes that can lead to cancer.

The Evidence So Far

A number of studies point to an association between antioxidants and a reduced cancer risk. The American Institute of Cancer Research [AICR] has funded dozens of these studies. Some results have shown:

- Vitamin C [in foods such as oranges and broccoli] may help reduce the risk of stomach cancer.
- Vitamin E [in foods such as almonds and whole wheat] may help lower the incidence of cancers of the prostate and colon.
- The mineral selenium [in mushrooms and whole grains] may reduce risk for prostate and lung cancers.
- Reservatrol, a phytochemical in red grapes, may inhibit growth of colon and other tumors, and help repair gene mutations.
- Whole grains contain a number of antioxidants that may help to protect the colon, where they become activated during the digestive process.

Researchers are becoming more convinced that cancer protection does not come from any single antioxidant. Dr. Ritva Butrum, Senior Science Advisor to AICR, says, "We seem to be past the stage of hoping that super-high doses of any one substance can be a 'magic bullet' against cancer or other health problems."

It will take more studies with human subjects to draw any firm conclusions about specific antioxidants. But enough evidence has accumulated to date so the general conclusion is quite clear: People who eat a mostly plant-based diet that contains plenty of fruits, vegetables, whole grains, beans and moderate amounts of nuts have lower cancer risk.

Some exciting research results show that within a few weeks of adding more fruits and vegetables to their diets, people who do not smoke have increased blood levels of antioxidants and decreased oxidative damage. This study also showed that one group that took supplements showed a reduction in oxidation damage, but still had more damage than the group that ate antioxidant-rich foods. An earlier study showed similar results.

Researchers have developed a test called "oxygen radical absorbance capacity" [ORAC] to determine the antioxidant capacity in specific vegetables, fruits and herbs. This test tube analysis measures the ORAC value in human blood. A higher score means greater effectiveness. Some results from ORAC studies so far are:

Food Item	Serving Size	ORAC Score
Pinto Beans	½ cup	11,864
Blueberry	1 cup	9,019
Cranberry	1 cup	8,983
Prune	½ cup	7,291
Strawberry	1 cup	5,938
Red Delicious Apples	1 whole	5,900

Other foods that showed high activity are kale, spinach, Brussels sprouts, broccoli, plums, oranges, red bell pepper and kiwi fruit, according to the USDA.

Why different foods appear to have more antioxidant capacity is not yet known, and may result from factors such as their genetic compositions. But the important thing to remember is that eating plenty and a wide variety of vegetables and fruits are the surest way to get the most antioxidant protection.

Future Directions for Antioxidant Research

Antioxidant researchers need to conduct more studies on how different antioxidants work in combination to affect cancer risk. It is known that these compounds interact with each other, influencing how effectively they are absorbed in the body.

In one recent study, rats fed a combination of tomato and broccoli powders made from whole vegetables showed significantly less prostate tumor growth than other groups of rats in the study that were fed tomato powder alone, broccoli powder alone, or only a diet supplemented with the isolated phytotchemical lycophene.

In fact, an increasing number of studies are showing that thousands of substances in plant foods seem to interact in complex ways. When some antioxidants are eaten together, some seem to reinforce and, in some cases, multiply each other's cancer fighting potential.

Scientists are now looking into how cooking and processing foods can increase or decrease the activity of some oxidants. Lycopene, for example, is absorbed more easily by the body when it is eaten in the form of processed tomato sauce and other products, rather than in the form of raw tomatoes.

Immune response also may be boosted by antioxidants, as some research suggests, which could help to promote health in many ways. Different antioxidants may be more effective than others against particular forms of cancer.

The very new field of research called "nutrigenomics" may actually someday be able to link an individual's genetic makeup with specific dietary substances, including antioxidants, to possibly help that person avoid diseases like cancer. Researchers funded by AIRC are working on finding answers like these.

Today's Message: Rely on Whole Foods

Researchers are beginning to understand how antioxidants work and can best be used. But experts at AICR believe that a diet rich in citrus, tomatoes, peppers, berries, grapes, broccoli, cabbage, greens like spinach and other vegetables, and fruits should provide all the antioxidants we need for good health and lower cancer risk.

For lower cancer risk, the American Institute for Cancer Research recommends filling 2/3 or more of your plate with plant-based foods like vegetables, fruit, whole grains and beans and 1/3 or less with animal proteins such as lean meat or dairy foods.

"The easiest advice is to cut down on animal products and eat a diet that is mostly made up of many brightly colored vegetables and fruits, along with whole grains and beans," says Dr. Butrum. "So many health protectors are naturally found in these foods that scientists estimate eating a large variety every day may lower cancer risk by at least 20 percent." Also, by getting regular physical activity and maintaining a healthy weight, leading cancer scientists say that people may lower their cancer risk even more by 30-40 percent.

Source: [Abstract] – American Institute for Cancer Research

If this chapter has stimulated your curiosity in what your body's antioxidant levels are, pay special attention to the paragraph on lipid peroxides in chapter 20.

Beware of Misleading Antioxidant Claims!

Nutritional supplement manufacturers are jumping on the free media exposure on the benefits of antioxidants. The manufacturers are exploiting every nutrient and any nutrient as a good source of antioxidants – which is not the case.

Note: This chapter or any other chapter in this book is not meant to dispense medical advice or strategies for your health care. It is meant to raise your awareness to be pro-active to other health options which should be discussed with your health care professional.

CHAPTER 9

My Favorite Nutritional Supplements and Fiber for My Heart and Circulation

    A.   L-Arginine
    B.   Beta-Carotene
    C.   B Vitamins
    D.   Vitamin C
    E.   Calcium
    F.   L-Carnitine
    G.   Vitamin E
    H.   Fiber
    I.   Garlic
    J.   Omega-3 Fish Oil
    K.   Magnesium
    L.   Quercitine
    M.   Coenzyme Q10 [CoQ10}

L-Arginine

L-Arginine, more commonly referred to simply as arginine, is an amino acid which has enormous effects on health of the endothelium [lining of the arteries]. It was in the early 1990's that scientists discovered that arginine is essential in the production of nitric oxide in the endothelium that keeps the arteries flexible and elastic doctors call "compliant." Literally, thousands of papers have been written in medical literature on the importance of nitric oxide and arginine.

Compliant arteries are capable of expanding to allow for whatever amount of flow the body requires. Noncompliant arteries gradually stiffen, losing their elasticity and dilate to accommodate that blood flow. The results are insufficient blood supplying body's tissues, increase in blood pressure and eventually hypertension.

Arginine production of nitric oxide performs the vital duty of its role as a vasodilator, meaning it helps control blood flow to every part of the body. Another key role of nitric oxide is to slow the accumulation of plaque in the blood. Arginine is not only safe when combined with statins, but also enhances the drugs' effect because one of the important mechanisms of these drugs is to increase and maintain nitric oxide production.

Source: Dr. Louis J. Ignarro, Nobel Laureate in Medicine.
Author of: *No More Heart Disease*

Beta-Carotene

Beta-carotene is the preferred form of Vitamin A because it does not have the same toxicity potential of Vitamin A.

What it can do for you:

- Shown to be preventative for certain types of cancer.
- Helpful in lowering levels of harmful cholesterol.
- A significant factor in <u>reducing the risks of heart disease</u>.
- Counteracts night blindness, weak eyesight, and aid in the treatment of many eye disorders. [It permits formation of visual purple in the eye.]
- Builds resistance to respiratory infections.
- Aids in the proper function of the immune system.
- Shortens the duration of diseases.
- Keeps the outer layer of your tissues and organs healthy.
- Helps in the removal of age spots.
- Promotes growth, strong bones, healthy skin, hair, teeth, and gums.
- Helps treat acne, superficial wrinkles, impetigo, boils, carbuncles, and open ulcers when applied externally.
- Aids in the treatment of emphysema and hyperthyroidism.

<u>Best Natural Source</u>:

Fish liver oil, liver, carrots, dark green and yellow vegetables, eggs, milk and dairy products, margarine, and yellow fruits. [Note: The color intensity of a fruit or vegetable is not necessarily a reliable indicator of its provitamin A content.]

B Vitamins

Like all the B-complex vitamins, any excess is created and not stored in the body. It is measured in milligrams [mg.].

Being synergistic, B vitamins are more potent together than when used separately. B1, B2, and B6 should be equally balanced [i.e., 50 mg. of B1, 50 mg. of B2, and 50 mg. of B6] to work effectively.

The official RDA for adults is 1.0 to 1.5 mg. [During pregnancy and lactation, 1.5 to 1.6 mg. is suggested.] Need increases during illness, stress, and surgery.

It is known as the "morale vitamin" because of its beneficial effects on the nervous system and mental attitude.

It has a mild diuretic effect.

<u>What it can do for you</u>:

- Promotes growth.
- Aids digestion, especially of carbohydrates.
- Improves your mental attitude.
- Keeps nervous system, muscles, and heart functioning normally.

- Helps fight air or seasickness.
- Relieves dental postoperative pain.
- Aids in treatment of herpes zoster.

Best Natural Sources:

Brewer's yeast, rice husks, unrefined cereal grains, whole wheat, oatmeal, peanuts, organic meats, lean pork, most vegetables, bran and milk.

Source: Earl Mindell's *Vitamin Bible*.

Vitamin C – A Water-Soluble Vitamin-Antioxidant

- Getting enough vitamin C may lower your risk of developing certain types of cancer.
- A combination of vitamin C, vitamin D, vitamin K, magnesium and phosphorus protects your bones against fractures.
  Source: Harvard Medical School, *The Benefits and Risks of Vitamins and Minerals*, SR 12000.
- It is essential to the development and maintenance of scar tissue, blood vessels and cartilage.

Source: Wikipedia.

Plays a primary role in the formation, which is important for growth and repair of body tissue cells, gums, blood vessels, bones and teeth.

- Helps in the body's absorption of iron.
- Lowers incidence of blood clots in veins.
- Prevents scurvy.
- Accelerates healing after surgery.

Best natural sources: citrus fruits, green and leafy vegetables, tomatoes, cauliflower, potatoes and peppers.

The best form vitamin C supplements containing complete C complex or bioflavonoids, hesperidem and rutin.

Daily doses most often used: 500 mg to 4 grams.

Toxicity: excessive intake can cause oxalic acid and uric acid stone formation, diarrhea, excessive urination and skin rashes.

Source: Earl Mindell's *Vitamin Bible*.

It helps support your adrenal glands and your immune system during stress.

There has also been good evidence that those with higher vitamin C levels excrete more heavy metals such as lead and mercury.

Source: *Ultra Metabolism*, Mark Hughman, M.D. Researches at Johns Hopkins have determined that a combination of vitamin C, Beta Carotene, Zinc oxide and copper can slow down macular degeneration.

Source: Dr. Isadore Rosenfeld, 2005. *Breakthrough Health*, Isadore Rosenfeld, M.D.

Calcium

There is more calcium in the body than any other mineral. Calcium and phosphorus work together for healthy bones and teeth. Calcium and magnesium work together for cardiovascular health.

Almost all of the body's calcium [two or three pounds] is found in the bones and teeth. Twenty percent of an adult's bone calcium is reabsorbed and replaced every year. [New bone cells form as old ones break down.] Calcium must exist in a two-to-one relationship with phosphorus [two parts calcium to one part phosphorus]. In order for calcium to be absorbed, the body must have sufficient vitamin D. For adults 800 to 1,200 mg. is the RDA. Calcium and iron are the two minerals most deficient in the American woman's diet.

What it can do for you:

- Alleviates insomnia.
- Helps metabolize your body's iron.
- Aids your nervous system, especially in impulse transmission.

On the cellular level, calcium is used to regulate the permeability and electrical properties of biological membranes [such as cell walls], which in turn control muscle and nerve functions, glandular secretions, and blood vessel dilation. Calcium is also essential for proper blood clotting. When calcium levels fall too low, nerve and muscle impairments can result. Skeletal muscles can spasm and the heart can beat abnormally – it can even cease functioning.

Best Natural Source:

Milk and milk products, all cheeses, soybeans, sardines, salmon, peanuts, walnuts, sunflower seeds, dried beans, kale, broccoli, collard greens.
Sources: Earl Mindell's *Vitamin Bible, http://www.faqs.org/nutrition/Ca-De/Calcium.html*

L-Carnitine

Numerous studies have shown that Co-Enzyme Q10 and L-carnitine help support a healthy heart and vascular function. L-carnitine is central to the body's ability to turn fat into energy. And any time you are trying to get a leaner physique, lower cholesterol, or lose weight, that's exactly what you want to do: turn fat into energy. There is no more natural way to support that process than with L-carnitine. Carnitine is a vitamin-like nutrient that occurs naturally in the body, but is found only in appreciable amounts in red meat. Its central role in helping cells make more energy is its lack of toxicity and its wide range of benefits. This has MADE IT A REMARKABLE NUTRIENT. People feel such an improved state of overall wellness and a natural increase in energy when they increase their intake of L-carnitine. Carnitine deficiency is more common than many people think, and can lead to such problems as overweight, fatigue, elevated triglycerides, and heart problems. Vegetarians often consume no L-carnitine in their diet, because L-carnitine is found predominantly only in foods of animal origin, such as red meat and milk. Fruits, vegetables, nuts and grains contain virtually none.

Source: [Abstract] – http://www.holistic2u.net/catalog/1_carnitine.htm

Vitamin E

What are the Different Forms of Vitamin E?

When reference is made to "Natural Vitamin E " it is called d-alpha tocopheryl acetate, or d-alpha tocopherol. If the name is preceded by dl – or just stated as alpha tocopheryl acetate or alpha tocopherol, then it is synthetic. Tocopherol [spelled with ol] means that the Vitamin E contains all four of the tocopherols [alpha, beta, gamma and delta] is the best and most effective form; if it is spelled with a yl, then it only contains alpha tocopheryl.

There are also four tocotrienols which will not be discussed in this format as all the research is not completed.

Vitamin E Protects Heart Health

Two Harvard Medical School studies reported a 47% reduction in risk of heart disease among nurses who had taken 200 IU of Vitamin E for more than two years, and a 37% lower risk of heart disease in men who had supplemented with 400 IU for more than two years.

Other studies suggest vitamin E improves:
- Immune function
- Brain function
- Eye function
- Lung function
- Protects against some cancers.

Any studies published in the *Journal of the American Medical Association* [*JAMA*] indicating vitamin E-alpha tocopherol by itself not to reduce heart attack factors were skewed because they did not do the studies with the therapeutic range of vitamin E; namely, alpha, beta, gamma and delta tocopherols.

Source: [Abstract] – Dr. Stephen Sinatra.

Fibers

Fiber's Critical Role

A century ago, before our food supply was industrialized and highly processed food became the norm, people ate an average of 28 grams of fiber a day. Conditions such as diabetes, heart disease, and obesity were far less common then than they are now. Even today, in cultures that eat a traditional, plant-based diet [sadly, there are fewer and fewer of them], diabetes, cancer, and cardiovascular disease are still rare. <u>By contrast, the United States currently ranks lowest in fiber intake and highest in deaths from heart disease among 20 developed nations.</u>

The 2003 European Prospective Investigation into Cancer and Nutrition, which spanned 10 countries and included 519,978 participants who were observed for nearly five years, found that those with the highest amounts of fiber in their diets had a 40% lower risk of developing colon cancer than those with the lowest fiber intake. <u>Other recent studies have found that increasing daily fiber intake by 10 grams lowers the risk of all coronary events by 14% and reduces the risk of death from heart disease by 27%. Fiber has been found to lower levels of triglycerides, low-density lipoprotein [LDL], C-reactive protein, and blood pressure – all of which are independent risk factors for heart attack and stroke.</u>

<u>Fiber Fights Metabolic Syndrome</u>

Another major risk factor for cardiovascular disease is body fat – particularly abdominal fat, which is strongly associated with elevated blood lipids, high blood pressure, and metabolic syndrome, a precursor to diabetes. High-fiber foods are digested much more slowly than are low-fiber foods, prolonging feelings of satiety or fullness by delaying the emptying of food from the stomach into the intestine, and allowing for the gradual absorption of nutrients from the small intestine into the bloodstream. This has significant implication for people with metabolic syndrome and diabetes. With the popularization of the glycemic index theory [which suggests minimizing the intake of foods that rapidly increase blood sugar], people with metabolic syndrome have been counseled to avoid starches and other carbohydrate-rich foods because it is believed that consuming them will lead to spikes in blood sugar and elevated insulin responses. This advice completely contradicts the latest scientific research.

For example, a recent article in the *Journal of Clinical Endocrinology & Metabolism* compared popular glycemic index-based, low-carbohydrate diets to a high-fiber, high carbohydrate diet emphasizing fresh fruits and vegetables. The study findings suggest that the fiber content of the foods eaten – rather than their glycemic index – was most beneficial for promoting insulin sensitivity. A classic Mediterranean diet, rich in carbohydrates and fiber from sources such as fruits, vegetables, whole grains, and nuts, has been shown over and over to be one of the best ways to improve metabolic syndrome. Because fiber slows the absorption of nutrients into the bloodstream, it naturally helps regulate blood sugar levels, preventing insulin surges and decreasing insulin resistance. I personally recommend eating two Metamucil wafers before each meal. They contain 6 grams of psyllium, a safe, well-tolerated fiber, which will slow absorption and help control insulin surges. It is abundantly clear that the best way to manage metabolic syndrome and decrease all of the cardiovascular risks that accompany it is by eating a diet high in complex carbohydrates supplying at least 25 grams of fiber a day.

<u>Fiber Promotes Weight Loss</u>

To help his patients lose weight and reduce their risk of heart disease and colon cancer, Dr. Schnue developed a program called the Reality Diet, which promotes cardiovascular health and weight loss through a high-fiber diet and exercise. Why high fiber? Research and clinical experience indicate that fiber is the single best predictor of success when it comes to weight loss.

First and foremost, fiber promotes satiety – in other words, it makes you feel satisfied or full. Satiety is one of the keys to successful weight loss, because no matter how much willpower you have, if your stomach is growling and you pass a Dunkin' Donuts, you will be hard pressed to resist. If you are completely full, however, you will have an easier time passing it by.

The federal government recommends that adults consume a minimum of 25 grams of fiber per day. On a good day, most Americans consume 12-17 grams. According to an article in the *Journal of the American Medical Association*, four popular fad diets – Atkins, Ornish, Weight Watchers, and Zone – provide an average of 15 grams per day. Yet study after study has shown that when people are allowed to eat as much as they want of a diet high in complex carbohydrates, they end up losing weight. Why? Because the fiber fills them up and they ultimately consume fewer calories per day.

Fiber may also help promote weight loss by preventing the absorption of calories from the intestine. A U.S. Department of Agriculture study showed that when a man doubled his fiber intake from 18 to 36 grams a day, he absorbed 130 fewer calories daily. Similarly, when a woman doubled her fiber intake from 12 to 24 grams a day, she absorbed 90 fewer calories daily. Over a year, that could add up to a weight loss of 9 pounds for women and more than 13 pounds for men.

Source: Dr. A. Schnue, South Florida Cardiology Associates.

Side Effects

Eating a large amount of fiber in a short period of time can cause intestinal gas [flatulence], bloating, and abdominal cramps. This usually goes away once the natural bacteria in the digestive system get used to the increase in fiber in the diet. Adding fiber gradually to the diet, instead of all at one time, can help reduce gas or diarrhea.

There are two types of fiber – soluble and insoluble. Both are important for health, digestion, and preventing diseases.
- Soluble fiber slows digestion and helps your body absorb vital nutrients from foods. It can be found in peas, beans and apples.
- Insoluble fiber adds bulk to the stool, helping foods pass more quickly through the stomach and intestines. It can be found in wheat bran.

The Bottom Line Recommendations for Fiber Intake

Fiber is an important part of a healthy diet, and you should get at least the minimum recommended amount of 10-25 grams of dietary fiber per day for adults. For children over age 2, the recommended intake is the child's age + 5 grams. The best sources are fresh fruits and vegetables, nuts, legumes, and whole-grain foods.

Some tips for increasing fiber intake:
- Eat whole fruits instead of drinking fruit juices.
- Replace white rice, bread, and pasta with brown rice and whole-grain products.
- Choose whole-grain cereals for breakfast.
- Snack on raw vegetables instead of chips, crackers, or chocolate bars.
- Substitute legumes for meat two or three times per week in chili and soups.
- Experiment with international dishes [such as Indian or Middle Eastern] that use whole grains and legumes as part of the main meal [as in Indian dahls] or in salads [for example, tabbouleh].

Sources:

Fuchs, C. S., Giovannucci, E. L., Colditz, G.A., et al. "Dietary fiber and the risk of colorectal cancer and adenoma in women." *New England Journal of Medicine*, 1999; 340:169-76.

Pereira, M. A., O'Reilly, E., Augustsson, K., et al. "Dietary fiber and risk of coronary heart disease: A pooled analysis of cohort studies." *Archive of Internal Medicine*, 2004; 164-370-6.

Van Horn, L.
Fiber, lipids, and coronary heart disease." A statement for healthcare professionals from the Nutrition Committee, American Heart Association.

Garlic

Garlic has been used as both food and medicine in many cultures for thousands of years, dating as far back as the time that the Egyptian pyramids were built. <u>Garlic is claimed to help prevent heart disease, including atherosclerosis</u>, high cholesterol, high blood pressure, and to improve the immune system. Garlic may also protect against cancer.

However, a rigorous NIH-funded clinical trial published by the "Archives of Internal Medicine," in February, 2007, found that consumption of garlic, in any form, did not reduce cholesterol levels in patients with moderately high levels.

With regard to this clinical trial, Heart.org reports, "Despite decades of research suggesting that garlic can improve cholesterol profiles, a new NIH-funded trial found absolutely no effects of raw garlic or garlic supplements on LDL, HDL, or triglycerides." The website says, "The findings underscore the hazards of meta-analysis made up of small, flawed studies and the value of rigorously studying popular herbal remedies." However, while garlic may not lower cholesterol levels in the bloodstream, <u>this study does not contradict studies that show that garlic protects arteries from that cholesterol</u>. For example, a Czech study found garlic supplementation reduced accumulation of cholesterol on vascular walls of animals. Another study had similar results, with garlic supplementation <u>significantly reducing the plaque in the aortas of cholesterol-fed rabbits</u>. Another study showed that supplementation with garlic extract inhibited vascular calcification in human patients with high blood cholesterol.

A study published in *Preventive Medicine* shows that garlic inhibits coronary artery calcification, a process that serves as a marker for plaque formation since the body lays down calcium in areas that have been damaged. In this year-long study, patients given aged garlic extract daily showed an average increase in their calcium score of 7.5%, while those in the placebo group had an average increase in calcium score of 22.2%.

Source: [Abstract] http://en.wikipedia.org/wiki/Garlic

Omega-3 Fish Oil

Omega-3 is from the Seas

Fish Oil is a natural source of Omega-3 fatty acids. Omega-3 fatty acids play a major role in cardiovascular health. Omega-3s also support the immune and nervous systems. Fish oil is vital for normal cell growth, and essential fatty acids play a key structural role in cell membranes. Fatty acids play a role in providing an energy source for the body, and may help support healthy joints.

Supplementation of Omega-3 fatty acids is most important since essential fatty acids cannot be made by the body and most Americans have low Omega-3 diets. The National Academy of Sciences, recognized as the highest scientific body in the U.S., recommends that men consume 1.6 grams and women consume 1.1 grams of Omega-3s per day. A balanced intake of Omega-3 and Omega-6 fatty acids is essential for good health.

A Fish Oil View of Heart Health

Two of the best-known Omega-3 fatty acids are EPA and DHA. Studies have shown that fish oil supplements containing EPA and DHA can support triglyceride health by helping to maintain levels already within a normal range. EPA is beneficial for circulation and makes more efficient use of oxygen for heart health maintenance. DHA also works to maintain healthy circulation.

Researchers performed two separate studies, one on women and one on men, to determine the effects of fish oil on heart health and healthy blood flow. In the study of men, supplementing with three grams of fish oil per day supported cholesterol health and also improved measures associated with smooth blood flow. In women, three grams of fish oil supported triglyceride health in younger subjects while supporting cholesterol health in older subjects.

All Omega-3 Fish oils are Not Equal
- Buy the highest quality available with GMP label [good manufacturing practices]. Also, check if the manufacturer has removed heavy metals, fat-soluble pollutants like PBCs and dioxins, and usually by molecular distillation.
- Most Omega-3 products list 1000 mg on the front label. That does not mean if you take two you are getting 2 grams of Omega-3 [1000 mg equals one gram].

If you look at the label on the back of the bottle, it will give you supplement facts of what comprises the 1000 mg. There you will see listed among other ingredients EPA and DHA [e.g., the Omega-3 I take has EPA 720 mg, DHA 480 mg = 1200 mg which converts to 1.2 grams.

The higher the actual EPA and DHA the product has will affect the price.

<u>What Exactly is an Omega Fat</u>?

Source: Ultra Prevention. Mark Hyman, M.D., Mark Lipons, M.D.

The omega classification refers to the chemical structure of unsaturated fats. Unsaturated fats are those that are generally liquids at room temperature, whereas predominantly saturated fats [such as butter] are solids at room temperature. [The omega numbers 3, 6, and 9 refer to the locations on the fat molecule where the hydrogen atom joins onto it. It is just basic chemical nomenclature, but these simple differences have profound biological effects in the body.]

For optimal health, bodies require a balance of omega fats. Deficiency of one or the other limits our ability to manufacture the full array of fats needed by our bodies for health cells, organs, and tissues. [Our bodies are normally about 15 to 30 percent fat by weight, depending on gender and body composition.]

Good sources of the omega-3 fats include: fish, flaxseed, omega-enriched eggs, organic canola oil, walnuts, brazil nuts, and sea vegetables. Good sources of the omega-6 oils include evening primrose oil, blackcurrant oil, borage oil, nuts, and seeds. Olive oil is the best source of the omega-9 fats—but don't forget avocados and nuts such as almonds.

- However, omega-6 fats are much more prevalent than omega-3 fats. The optimal ratio of omega-6 to omega-3 fats in our diet should be between 2:1 and 4:1, whereas the standard American diet has a ratio of more than 20:1. This means most of us need to increase our intake of omega-3 fats and reduce our intake of omega-6 fats. [Omega-9 foods generally play more of a role in our American Diet, whereas most of us should get the lion's share of our fats from omega-3s and omega-9s.]
- Of all of the fats, our bodies actually require only two: *alphalinoleic acid* [an omega-3] and *linoleic acid* [an omega-6]. As with some vitamins, our bodies need these two fats but cannot manufacture them. By using these as raw materials, however, we can manufacture all of the other fats our bodies use.

Sources of the omega-6 linoleic acid include safflower and sunflower oils, and corn, soy, and canola oils. Sources of the omega-3 alpha-linoleic acid include flaxseed oil and blackcurrant seed oil. They can also be found in smaller amounts in certain nuts and seeds.

<u>Earl Mendell's *Vitamin Bible* states what Omega-3 will do for you</u>.

- <u>Helps retard atherosclerosis</u>
- <u>Lowers LDL cholesterol and triglycerides</u>
- <u>Reduces blood viscosity and help prevent heart attacks and strokes</u>
- <u>Lowers blood pressure</u>
- <u>Enhances the immune system</u>
- <u>Alleviates rheumatoid arthritis</u>

- Helps protect the body from lupus erithematosus
- Offers protection against migraines and kidney disease

If you're a vegetarian, omega-3 fatty acids can also be found in vegetable oils such as soybean, canola and flaxseed—but the conversion to EPA and DHA is much slower.

Some Interesting Omega-3 Studies

- Additional support for fish oils comes from a report on nearly 80,000 women in the Nurses' Health Study. Published in 2001 in the *Journal of the American Medical Association*, this 14-year study found that eating fish at least twice a week versus less than once a month cut in half the risk of strokes caused by clots blocking an artery to the brain. The Nurses' Health Study also found that eating one to three servings of fish per month cut the risk of heart disease by 20% while eating at least five servings a week lowered risk by 40%.
  Source: Special Health Report from Harvard Medical School.

Stephen Sinatra, M.D. Published Three Studies in *Heart Sense* in April 2000 [Abstract]:

An Italian group of investigators, identified by the acronym "GISSI," recruited more than 11,000 participants for the study. Each of them had had a heart attack within three months of the study's inception. They were randomly assigned a diet consisting of fish oil [1 g/day], vitamin E [300 IU/day], a combination of both, or a placebo. There were about 2,750 participants in each of the four groups, and the study tracked them for an average of 3½ years.

The study findings were extremely impressive for fish oil. Here is a brief summary of what the fish-oil group experienced:

- A reduction in nonfatal myocardial infarction [MI], stroke, and death from all causes
- A decrease in total mortality
- A decrease in cardiovascular [CV] death
- A 17 percent decrease in sudden death

In contrast—and surprisingly—the findings were not very impressive for vitamin E. The people who took fish oil with vitamin E fared no better than those who took fish oil alone. What happened with vitamin E? Well, in spite of its powerful anti-oxidant, anti-cancer, and anti-aging capabilities, vitamin E just didn't show significant cardiovascular disease prevention capabilities in the GISSI study.

This contradiction between the GISSI findings and those of the 1996 Cambridge Heart Antioxidant Study [CHAOS] is very surprising. The CHAOS study is one of the most famous cardiology studies done to date. It showed a protective heart benefit for those who were taking about 400-800 IU of vitamin E daily [a higher dose than was taken by participants in the GISSI study]. The results of the CHOAS study have yet to be duplicated, so more research needs to be done before vitamin E's heart effects are fully known. But other studies have shown many other benefits from vitamin E, so its place in a healthy daily regimen is still assured.

Most of the research indicates that fish oil has several protective functions, including the following:

1. The inhibition of clotting events in blood vessels
2. The reduction of inflammation and, in turn, the risk of plaque rupture
3. A third benefit that results from the effects of the first two: should plaque rupture occur, the likelihood is *much* less that a clot will congeal and attach to the debris, cutting off blood flow entirely and causing a myocardial infarction.
4. The suppression of cardiac arrhythmias, often the precursors of sudden cardiac death

The GISSI team feels that the fourth benefit may be the most important, especially in terms of reducing cardiac deaths. You see, not only does fish oil penetrate plaque and help prevent plaque rupture; it also gets inside isolated cardiac cells.

Magnesium

Magnesium is essential to all living cells, and is the 11th most abundant element by mass in the human body.

Necessary for calcium and vitamin-C metabolism, as well as that of phosphorus, sodium, and potassium.
Measured in milligrams [mg.].
Essential for effective nerve and muscle functioning.
Important for converting blood sugar into energy.
Known as the anti-stress mineral.
Alcoholics are usually deficient.
The human body contains approximately 21 g. of magnesium.

What it can do for you

- Promotes a healthier cardiovascular system and help prevent heart attacks
- Keeps teeth healthier.
- Helps prevent calcium deposits, kidney and gallstones.
- Brings relief from indigestion.
- Combined with calcium can work as a natural tranquilizer.

Magnesium works best with vitamin A, calcium, and phosphorus.

Source: Earl Mindell's *Vitamin Bible*.

Quercetin

Quercetin is a flavonoid and, more specifically, a flavonol. It is the aglycone form of a number of other flavonoid glycosides, such as rutin and quercitrin found in citrus fruit. Quercetin is found to be the most active of the flavonoids in studies, and many medicinal plants owe much of their activity to their high quercetin content. Quercetin has demonstrated significant anti-inflammatory activity because of direct inhibition of several initial processes of inflammation. For example, it inhibits both the manufacture and release of histamine and other allergic/inflammatory mediators. In addition, it exerts potent antioxidant activity and vitamin C-sparing action.

Quercetin forms the glycosides quercetrin and rutin together with rhamnose and rutinose, respectively.

Quercetin also shows remarkable anti-tumor properties. A recent study in the *British Journal of Cancer* shows that when treated with a combination of quercetin and ultrasound at 20 KHz for 1 minute duration, skin and prostate cancers show a 90% mortality within 48 hours with no viable mortality of normal cells. Note that ultrasound also promotes topical absorption by up to 1,000 times making the use of topical quercetin and ultrasound wands an interesting proposition.

Quercetin may have positive effects in combating or helping to prevent cancer, prostatitis, heart disease, cataracts, allergies/inflammations, and respiratory diseases such as bronchitis and asthma.

Foods rich in quercetin include capers, lovage, apples, tea, onions, red grapes, citrus fruits, broccoli and other leafy green vegetables, cherries, and a number of berries including raspberries.

Source: [Abstract] http://en.wikipedia.org/wiki/Quercetin

Coenzyme Q 10 [CoQ10]

One of our bodies' best defenses against oxidative stress and chronic disease of aging is coenzyme Q 10 which your body manufactures. Unfortunately, as we get older, it manufactures less and less.

If you are on a statin drug [*which depletes it to an insufficient level*], you should be taking CoQ10. Your doctor will prescribe the proper dosage needed.

Coenzyme Q10 [CoQ10] is a fat soluble cofactor essential for energy producing metabolic pathways and for the proper functioning of the mitrochondrial oxidative system. With insufficient CoQ10, the electron transfer activity of the mitrochondria decrease, resulting in a net failure to produce the energy necessary to run the cell. Tissues with high energy demand have even greater demands for CoQ10. For example, the heart muscle, which continually exerts a pumping action for an entire lifetime, has an immense need for this cofactor. Studies demonstrate the effectiveness of supplemental coenzyme Q10 in cardiomyopathy, myocardial dysfunction and congestive heart failure. CoQ10 is also a powerful antioxidant like vitamins E and C and thus serves the role of neutralizing excess from radicals. It is now well established that the control of excessive free radical activity is key in preventing/delaying the progression of degenerative disease.

Source: Quest Diagnostic Labs, Dr. S. Sinatra [*yes, he is a cousin of Frank Sinatra*].

Note: This chapter or any other chapter in this book is not meant to dispense medical advice or strategies for your health care. It is meant to raise your awareness to be pro-active to other health options which should be discussed with your health care professional.

CHAPTER 10

Introduction to Nine Silent Assailants

I have selected my personal favorites which are not suggesting medical priority of one over the other. I call them:

Headliners

Elevated cholesterol, low HDL, elevated LDL and elevated triglycerides.

Byliners

C-reactive protein, elevated homocysteine, elevated glucose.

Rear Page

Last but not least, blood viscosity and hypertension

Before we venture into the 9 silent assailants threatening your heart, I would like you to consider your heredity. It typically determines 30% of your lifespan. Then your genes will contribute to more than 30% of your life span.

That means to the majority of us that the other 70% of our lifespan is controlled by our lifestyle and environment according to Thomas Perls, M.D., MPH Director of Boston University's New England Centenarian study.

There is a place for you between being a gym rat and a couch potato.

The following newsletters as well as numerous books on health, and study after study that I have researched , all advocate exercise as your #1 priority [and if you smoke, STOP], which supports and strengthens your cardiovascular system and, therefore, your entire well-being, which will allow you to enjoy your life and family.

- Johns Hopkins Health After 50
- Harvard Heart Letter
- Duke Medicine Health Letter
- University of California Berkley Wellness Letter
- Cleveland Clinic Heart Letter
- Tufts University Health Letter
- Consumers Reports, on Health
- Life Extension Magazine
- Dr. Stephen Sinatra, Heart, Health and Nutrition

If you were to ask your traditional medicine doctor, "Doc, what can I do to avoid a heart problem," he would say "stop smoking, lose weight, exercise, eat right and so on"

As far as eating right, it's next to impossible to get the proper nutrition from the food you eat due to soil depletion caused by lack of proper crop rotations. Our so-called authority on nutrition, the FDA and their experts keep changing the food pyramid. It's a very inexpensive insurance policy to consider nutrition supplements in addition to trying to eat a proper diet.

Let's face it; your doctor is not going to be your personal trainer. You have to be your own health advocate. There are many factors contributing to heart and arterial complications.

Bypass the Bypass

If you are reading this book, you have contemplated or are contemplating being your own health advocate either because you or a loved one or a friend have experienced great disillusionments with health care and advice provided by your or their doctors.

Bypasses, angioplasty, and stents are strictly a band-aid remedy. In most cases they were required because your heart and arterial system has disintegrated.

In most cases, these procedures were performed in an emergency situation and you were left with two choices by your doctors—the procedure or almost certain death. There really was only one choice you could make.

After this procedure it's a rare doctor who will take the time to tell you how lucky you were and to also tell you this was not a cure. It could happen again. You must change your lifestyle and then proceed to give yourself a strategy to do so.

Dr. William B. Stason of Brandeis University, author of an article in the October 2007 *Journal of Circulation* states: "Bypass surgery and artery cleaning procedures don't actually cure the patient. They only address the most pressing symptoms of heart disease. It takes lifestyle changes and medications to fix the underlying problem."

Hopefully, this book will heighten your awareness that there is more than one option than the emergency room to improve your heart and its arterial system.

Be Good to Your Heart, and Your Arterial System,
Your Most Dependable Friend

Heart Facts

- Hold out your hand and make a fist. If you're a kid, your heart is about the same size as your first, and if you're an adult, it's about the same size as two fists.
- The heart pumps about 1 million barrels of blood during an average lifetime—that's enough to fill more than 3 super tankers.
- Your heart beats about 100,000 times in one day and about 35 million times in a year. During an average lifetime, the human heart will beat more than 2.5 billion times.
- Give a tennis ball a good, hard squeeze. You're using about the same amount of force your heart uses to pump blood out to the body. Even at rest, the muscles of the heart work hard—twice as hard as the leg muscles of a person sprinting.

- Feel your pulse by placing two fingers at pulse points on your neck or wrists. The pulse you feel is blood stopping and starting as it moves through your arteries. As a kid, your resting pulse might range from 90 to 120 beats per minute. As an adult, your pulse rate slows to an average of 72 beats per minute.
- The aorta, the largest artery in the body, is almost the diameter of a garden hose. Capillaries, on the other hand, are so small that it takes ten of them to equal the thickness of a human hair.
- Relative total length of veins, arteries and capillaries: There are no actual measurements available. But the reported estimate is 100,000 miles for an average adult.
- Your body has about 5.6 liters [6 quarts] of blood. These 5.6 liters of blood circulate through the body three times every minute. In one day, the blood travels a total of 19,000 km [12,000 miles]—that's four times the distance across the U.S.

Source: Thirteen W.E.N.T. N.Y.

"Heart Speak: The many Meanings of 'Heart Disease'

When it comes to matters of the heart, clinical terms require careful consideration so that you know which recommendations apply to you. Here's a list of common conditions that fall under the broad category of 'heart disease.'

Acute Coronary Syndrome: A term used to describe conditions ranging from unstable angina to heart attack, which suddenly reduce blood flow to the heart.

Angina: Chest pain that results when atherosclerosis narrows coronary arteries to limit the supply of oxygen and blood to the heart.

Arrhythmia: An irregular or abnormal heart beat.

Atherosclerosis: Atherosclerosis is the underlying cause of heart disease in most people. It occurs when fatty deposits [plaques] build up within walls of the coronary arteries. [Atherosclerosis and arteriosclerosis both refer to the same abnormality.]

Cardiac Arrest: An abrupt loss of the heart's ability to pump blood, usually due to a heart rhythm abnormality. [Cardiac arrest is not the same as a heart attack.]

Cardiovascular Disease [CVD]: CVD refers to any disease that reduces the blood supply from the arteries to the heart and other organs. The most common examples of CVD are coronary heart disease, peripheral artery disease, and cerebrovascular disease.

Congenital Heart Disease: "Congenital" means present at birth. This form of heart disease is an abnormality in the structure or function of the heart that develops before birth.

Coronary Heart Disease [CHD]: CHD occurs when the arteries that supply blood to the heart are narrowed by the buildup of plaque [atherosclerosis]. CHD is also referred to as coronary artery disease [CAD].

Heart Failure: Heart failure occurs when the heart is unable to pump enough blood to meet the body's needs.

Hypertension: Chronic hypertension, or high blood pressure, can lead to heart failure, stroke, and kidney disease by increasing the demands on the heart.

Myocardial Infarction: Commonly known as heart attack, a myocardial infarction occurs when a blood clot at the site of a plaque in a coronary artery blocks blood flow to a portion of the heart and results in death of heart muscle.

Myocarditis, Endocarditis, or Pericarditis: Acute inflammation of the myocardium [heart muscle], pericardium [the membrane surrounding the heart], or endocardium [the inner lining of the heart]."

Source: Johns Hopkins Medical Letter, 11/07.

"Midlife Risk Factors May Predict Men's Length and Quality of Life

Men who avoid certain risk factors in midlife are more likely to live longer, healthier lives, suggests a study in the November 15th issue of the *Journal of the American Medical Association.* For up to 40 years, researchers followed 5,820 Japanese-American men, age 45-68, who were free of illness and functional impairments at the start of the study. Of those patients, 2,451 survived to age 85, and 655 of them met criteria for "exceptional survival," or living to a specific age without developing physical or cognitive impairment and six major chronic diseases: heart disease, cancer [excluding melanoma skin cancer], stroke, Parkinson's disease, chronic obstructive pulmonary disease [COPD] and treated diabetes. The men who in mid-life avoided risk factors such as smoking, excessive drinking, high blood pressure, high blood sugar, high triglycerides [a type of fat in the body] and being overweight were more likely to live longer and live exceptionally, the researchers reported. They calculated that men with no midlife risk factors had a 69 percent likelihood they would survive to age 85, and that figure dropped to as low as 22 percent for men with six or more risk factors. Also, men with no risk factors had a 55 percent probability they would live exceptionally to age 85, compared with a 9 percent likelihood for those with six or more risk factors, the study suggested.

Wellness Facts

- The death rate from heart disease was cut in half between 1980 and 2000 in the U.S. This saved an estimated 342,000 lives in 2000 alone. About 44% of these lives were saved by preventive measures, notably reducing blood pressure and cholesterol and stopping smoking, concludes a new analysis in the new *England Journal of Medicine*. The rest were saved by improved treatments for those with heart disease.

Talk about Irony.

While I was still in research for this book, I came across an article in the "LI Business" section of *Newsday* on 10/24/07. "South Nassau Communities Hospital in Oceanside, New York is adding a 32,000 square foot Facility to their 441 Bed Hospital."

Guess what it's for.

It is to do angioplasty. That's a procedure doctors use to unclog blocked arteries.

If you don't want to become a patient in a similar facility, please take heed and take away some of the information I am writing about in this book.

Note: This chapter or any other chapter in this book is not meant to dispense medical advice or strategies for your health care. It is meant to raise your awareness to be pro-active to other health options which should be discussed with your health care professional.

CHAPTER 11

Elevated Cholesterol Spear

Understanding Cholesterol will Improve your Health

We have all heard about cholesterol. Advertisers promote their low cholesterol products: low fat ice cream, fat free milk, etc. But how many of us really understand cholesterol? *There is good fat and bad fat; high density and low density*, etc. What does all that mean and how does it impact our health? Let's take a look at cholesterol and how it impacts our dietary choices and our health. Understanding cholesterol is the key to a healthy diet.

What is Cholesterol?

The total cholesterol number on your lab report is comprised of your HDL, LDL, VLDL and triglycerides. However, if you total the HDL, LDL, VLDL and triglycerides, they will exceed your total cholesterol number. The lab has a formula to complete that total cholesterol number.

Cholesterol is a fat-like substance produced primarily in our liver but also found in the foods we eat. The body makes all the cholesterol we need but what exactly do we need cholesterol for? In fact, cholesterol has several important functions including:
- the formation and maintenance of cell membranes
- the formation of sex hormones
- the production of bile salts that help digest foods
- the production of Vitamin D

If We Need Them, Why Are We Concerned About Having Too Much?

As part of your routine care, your doctor will often perform a blood test that measures the amount of cholesterol in your blood. For some, the levels are just right. But for many, their diet, the medications they take, or their genetic make-up, causes their levels of cholesterol to be higher than required by the body. Unfortunately, more is not better. In fact, having too much cholesterol in your blood can be a threat to your health. Higher than normal levels of cholesterol have been linked to:
- heart disease characterized by chest pain and heart attacks
- peripheral vascular disease (clogged arteries in the legs)
- stroke as a result of clogged arteries in the head and neck
- pancreatitis and lipodystrophy

Not All Fats Are Bad

While too much fat is bad for your health, there are types of fat that are actually better for you than others. In fact, some fats have been shown to decrease your risk of heart disease. It is important to know which are the "good fats" and which are the "bad fats." *(See tips from Heart Association for good and bad fats, and Dr. Dr. Sinatra's recommendations, as you read on.)*

American Heart Association Recommendations

Total Cholesterol Level	Category
Less than 200 mg/dL	Desirable
200-239 mg/dL	Borderline High
240 mg/dL and above	High

*Cholesterol levels are measured in milligrams (mg) of cholesterol per deciliter (dL) of blood.

In the past, it was thought to be good enough to have a cholesterol level better than average. Until recently, doctors advised their patients to strive for a total cholesterol lower than 200 mg/dL. Eventually, this advice was to be lacking and now we know that it is not very good to be average in a population that ubiquitously develops atherosclerosis. When autopsies were performed, almost all American adults demonstrate significant coronary artery disease (and even 78% of young trauma victims who died before the age of 35 demonstrated significant atherosclerosis on autopsy. If you eat American food, you will inevitably develop American diseases. It is rare that someone can escape from the biological laws of cause and effect.

Clearly, if we attempt to rival the low cholesterol of populations that eat mostly natural plant foods and do not have heart disease, we are always looking at total cholesterols below 150 mg/dL. The average cholesterol level in rural China, as documented in the massive China Cornell Project, was 127 mg/dL. Heart attacks were rare, and both cancer and heart disease rates plummeted as cholesterol levels fell, which reflected very low animal product consumption. The lowest occurrence of heart disease and cancer occurred in the group that consumed plant-based diets with less than two servings of animal products per week.

Here are some tips for lowering your overall cholesterol, from the American Heart Association:

- Eat fewer than 30 percent calories from fat. Dr. Dean Ornish, author of *Reversing Heart Disease*, recommends as little as 10 percent calories from fat.
- Choose polyunsaturates – such as safflower, sesame and sunflower seeds, corn and soybeans – and monounsaturates – such as canola, olive and peanut oils and avocados.
- Eat less than 10 percent calories from saturated fat, such as butter, lard and tropical oils including coconut and palm.
- Other foods high in saturated fat include beef, veal, lamb, pork, poultry [dark meat and skin] fat, cream, milk and cheese. These foods also are high in cholesterol.
- Consume no more than 300 milligrams cholesterol daily.
- Eat no more than four egg yolks a week. One egg yolk contains about 213 milligrams cholesterol. Egg whites do not contain cholesterol.
- Eat fish, poultry without skin and lean meats. Use low-fat or skim dairy products.
- Consider that shrimp and crayfish are higher in cholesterol than most fish, but lower in fat and saturated fat than most meats and poultry.
- Avoid processed meats, such as sausage, bologna, salami and hot dogs. About 70 to 80 percent of their calories came from fat.
- Buy "choice" or "select" grades of beef, instead of "prime." Read labels.
- Trim fat from meat before cooking. Use a rack to drain fat when broiling, roasting or baking.

- Hamburger adds more fat to the American diet than any other food.
- Broil rather than pan-fry meats such as hamburger and steak.
- Other cooking methods that require little or no fat are boiling, poaching, steaming, sautéing and microwaving.
- Occasionally snack on nuts and seeds. Though high in fat and calories, most of the fat is unsaturated. Nuts and seeds contain protein, but no cholesterol.
- Choose complex carbohydrates for about 50 percent of your daily calories. They include whole grains, fresh fruits and vegetables, beans, rice and pasta. Many of these foods are high in fiber, which helps flush our bodies of "bad" LDL cholesterol.
- Starting at age 20, have your total cholesterol and HDL checked.
- Exercise, maintain a healthy weight and quit smoking.

For more information about cholesterol, call the American Heart Association toll-free hotline: 1 (800) HEARTLINE.

Source: American Heart Association.

The Innocuous (Harmless) High Fructose Corn Syrup (HFCS)

This is really a wolf in lamb's clothing. (Abstracted and edited from Mark Hyman, M.D., author of *Ultra Metabolism*).

High fructose corn syrup is probably the biggest reason for the increase in cholesterol levels we have seen in our society over the last 20 years. This isn't such a problem when you eat fructose the way nature intended it to be eaten, in the form of fruit. This is because when you eat fruit, the amount of fructose you ingest is significantly lower than in sweetened beverages, and the metabolic effects of it are different because the increased intake of fiber, vitamins, minerals, phytonutrients, and antioxidants helps slow absorption and improve metabolism.

However, when fructose is processed into high-fructose corn syrup (HFCS), it is absorbed more quickly than regular sugar and enters your cells without any help. It doesn't require the help of insulin the way glucose does. Once inside the cell, it becomes an uncontrolled source of carbon (acetyl-CoA) that is then made into Cholesterol and triglycerides. <u>Basically, that means that eating HFCS makes your cholesterol level shoot straight up and causes problems with your liver that slow down your metabolism even more</u>. It actually produces a fatty liver (just like foie gras or pâté) and is the major cause of abnormal liver function tests in this country.

Corn syrup does not have the same recognition, which is very surprising to me, perhaps because it doesn't appear as much on labels as HFCS. But folks, they have the same effect when eaten.

If you start to read ingredients on the rear label – don't be fooled by statements on the product's front label such as: "All natural or fat free."

If you check your refrigerator or pantry, and of course, your supermarket, you'll find these syrups are used by commercial food manufacturers in just about every processed food you find in the U.S. today: cereals, Graham crackers, cereal bars, salad dressings, all maple syrups –

except pure Vermont Maple Syrup, Ketchup, other condiments, ice creams, breads, soft drinks, prepackaged meals and fast foods. It's almost ubiquitous.

Fiber and Heart Disease

In the United States, coronary heart disease is a leading cause of death for both men and women. This disease is characterized by a buildup of <u>cholesterol-filled plaque in the coronary arteries</u> – the arteries that feed the heart. This causes them to become hard and narrow, a process referred to as atherosclerosis. Total blockage of a coronary artery produces a heart attack.

High intake of dietary fiber has been linked to a lower risk of heart disease in a number of large studies that followed people for many years. In a Harvard study of over 40,000 male health professionals, researchers found that a high total dietary fiber intake was linked to a 40 percent lower risk of coronary heart disease, compared to a low fiber intake. Cereal fiber, the fiber found in grains, seemed particularly beneficial. A related Harvard study of female nurses produced quite similar findings.

Source: Harvard School of Public Health.

Partial List of Fruits and Vegetables and Their Fiber Amount in Grams per Day
(Bear in mind, your ideal target is 30 to 35 grams per day.
[All values are from *Family Circle Magazine*])

<u>Fruits</u>

Apples	2.5 grams	
Apricots	2.2	"
Bananas	2.1	"
Blueberries ½ c.	2.5	"
Cantaloupe ½ c.	2.7	"
Cherries ½ c.	1.7	
Figs – one	3.7	"
Grapefruit – med.	1.7	"
Orange	1.6	"
Peach	1.6	"
Pear	5	"
Pineapple ½ c.	1.2	"
Plum	1.4	"

<u>Vegetables</u>

Asparagus – 6 spears	2.2 grams	
Beans (Snap) ½ c.	2.1	"
Beets ½ c.	2.2	"
Beans (Lima) ½ c.	4.4	"
Broccoli 1- spear	4.5	"
Cabbage ½ c.	2	"
Carrots, raw – 1 med.	2.4	"
Cauliflower ½ c.	1.4	"
Corn, yellow	2.9	"
Lettuce, leaf 1 c.	1.2	"
Onion ½ c.	2.6	"
Peas, green ½ c.	4.1	"
Potato, baked	3.7	"
Spinach ½ c.	2.1	"
Squash, winter ½ c.	3.4	"
Sweet Potato ½ c.	3.8	"
Tomato 1 med	1.0	"
Zucchini ½ c.	2.7	"

<u>Some High Fiber Cereals and Wafers</u>

Quaker Oats ½ c.	4 grams	
Kellogg's Mueslix ⅔ c.	4	"
Kellogg's Mini Wheats ¾ c.	5	"

Quaker Raison Bran 1 ¼ c.	6	"
Grainfields Whole Grain Raisin Bran	7	"
Metamucil Fiber – 2 wafers to a package; 12 to a box (contains psyllium)	6	"

Psyllium Husk

<u>Psyllium seed husk may reduce the risk of heart disease by lowering cholesterol levels</u>, and is known to help alleviate the symptoms of irritable bowel syndrome, though it often causes uncomfortable bloating. Psyllium husk may be used as a bulk-forming laxative.

Dr. David W. Tanton, Ph.D., author of *Drug-Free Approach to Health Care* (abstracted).

Strengthen your Thyroid. A low thyroid condition will often result in elevated cholesterol. In fact, elevated cholesterol was once used as an indicator that a hypothyroid (low thyroid) condition might exist.

Flax Seed Oil. An article in the October 2002 issue of the *Health Alert* newsletter stated that if you have abnormally high cholesterol levels, take at least one tablespoon of raw flax oil daily. This may be one of the most profound ways to normalize cholesterol. A flax oil study was reported in an editorial in the medical journal *Circulation*, February 16, 1999, showing that people consuming flax oil daily enjoyed a 70% reduction in deaths from heart disease compared to those not getting the oil. Incidentally, flax oil is inexpensive and readily available, and is often beneficial in resolving depression also.

Policosanol. The American Council on Collaborative Medicine published the following information (*ACCM Health Sense*, July 2003):

"Policosanol Inhibits Cholesterol Synthesis

A waxy long-chain alcohol derived from Caribbean sugar cane, policosanol is not considered a sugar molecule, thus is safe for diabetics. <u>One of the newest discoveries for controlling cholesterol</u>, 14 separate studies show policosanol not only lowers total cholesterol by significant margins, but reduces LDL up to 29% while increasing HDL by 8-15%.

Research shows it is also considered equally as effective as statin drugs (such as Lipitor™) for normalizing cholesterol levels, thus avoids common side effects like muscle atrophy and liver dysfunction."

Vitalzyme™. According to Dr. William Wong, N.D., the natural protolytic (protein digesting) enzyme, <u>Vitalzyme™ has been found to reduce cholesterol levels by 21% in only 3 weeks</u>. He attributes the action to the fat digesting enzyme (lipase) in the formula. Although the protein-digesting enzyme (protease) also found in the formula won't likely have an influence on cholesterol, it will remove the fibrin in the arteries that can contribute to the restriction of blood flow. This can help prevent the clotting that often results in heart attacks or strokes, our primary objective.

Niacin (vitamin B₃) is proven to lower cholesterol and to improve circulation. Niacin also assists in the metabolism of both carbohydrates and fats, and cholesterol is a fat. High doses of the non-flushing form of niacin are highly effective in removing cholesterol, although regarding some people, long-term use can sometimes result in liver inflammation. If so, the problem can be easily eliminated simply by discontinuing its use. Niacin is commonly depleted by alcohol, antibiotics, caffeine, and SSRI antidepressants, as well as stress.

The omega-3 fatty acid DHA, derived from fish oil, not only helps thin the blood, but also lowers both the blood pressure and <u>cholesterol levels</u>, all important for our overall cardiovascular health, although it can easily be depleted by both estrogen and oral contraceptives.

Large doses of vitamins C lowers cholesterol levels and prevents oxidization of cholesterol as well as lowering high blood pressure. It also aids in the production of anti-stress hormones. Vitamin C is commonly depleted by sugar, alcohol, caffeine, antidepressants, contraceptives, but especially smoking. An increased level of <u>vitamin C assists in the conversion of cholesterol to bile acids, which promotes the digestion of fats, and the removal of excess cholesterol</u>.

Guggul. Documentation shows that the herb known as <u>guggul outperforms prescription pharmaceuticals in the reduction of total cholesterol</u>, lowering triglycerides and increasing the HDL level. As stated in the July 2003 *Health Sense* Nutritional Supplement, published by the American Council on Collaborative Medicine, Inc. (ACCM), in one study, 20 patients with high cholesterol were given guggul two times a day for 16 weeks, resulting in cholesterol levels that dropped 22%, triglycerides down 27% and HDL up by 36%. Another study showed it reduced the tendency of blood to clot by 30-40% in patients with coronary heart disease.

Dr. Stephen Sinatra of *Heart Sense* recommends:

"A Natural Cholesterol-Lowering Remedy

If you're among the millions of Americans struggling with elevated cholesterol, you can tackle it with plant sterols. You don't have to settle for cholesterol-lowering drugs (statins) unless you have advanced heart disease.

How Phytosterols Work

Phytosterols work primarily by inhibiting the body's ability to absorb dietary cholesterol. Some research suggests that phytosterols also inhibit the body's reabsorption of cholesterol secreted into the bile, but this research is still inconclusive.

If you take phytosterol supplements, I recommend 75-100 mg either before or during each meal. Your health food store will typically carry these supplements. "

Source: Dr. Stephen Sinatra, *Heart Sense.*

ProFibe *[abstracted from ProFibe literature]* – The medical community has been aware of the ability of water soluble dietary fibers [WSF] to naturally lower blood cholesterol LDL levels in humans.

• Developed at the University of Florida by Dr. James Cerda and Charles Burgin, ProFibe is a patented, award-winning formula consisting of guar gum and citrus pectin complexed to non-GMOs [genetically modified] by protein. The result? A water soluble fiber supplement which is 100% usable by the body.

Usable water soluble fiber [WSF] can dramatically reduce cholesterol [LDL-C] levels by as much as 25-30% in one month! Other benefits may include reduced atherosclerosis, better digestion, improved glucose tolerance, weight loss and lowered blood pressure. Many ProFibe users report enhanced energy levels as well.

• **Case Study I**
A 58 year-old white male taking 10 mg of Zocor one/day. His total cholesterol was 221. His LDL-C was 137 and his triglycerides were 243. ProFibe was introduced at three servings per day with the 10 mg of Zocor, for 30 days. At the end of the 30 days the subject's total cholesterol was 159, LDL-C was 86 and the triglycerides were 187. The risk factor improved from 3.9 to 2.4.

• **Case Study II**
A 53 year-old white female taking 10 mg of Zocor per day. Her total cholesterol of 249, her LDL-C was 158 and her triglycerides were 198. At the end of 30 days of taking three servings per day of ProFibe with the 10 mg of Zocor, the total cholesterol was 216, LDL-C was 134 and triglycerides were 130. Risk factor improved from 3.1 to 2.4.

• **Case Study III**
A 61 year-old white female with a recent history of CAD. Taking 20 mg per day of Mevacor, she had a total cholesterol of 301, and an LDL-C of 141. After taking three servings per day of ProFibe with the Mevacor for only 14 days, the total cholesterol dropped to 217 and the LDL-C fell to 84. The risk factor dropped from 4.7 to 3.2.

Not only is ProFibe™ safe and proven effective, it is easy to use. Three servings a day are recommended, which supply us a whopping 18 mg of fiber, over one-half of the daily recommended amount. This provides as much beneficial WSF as a bucket of oatmeal, a dozen oranges or a bushel of apples! Yet you cannot receive the same healthy benefits from fruit alone or other supplements on the market. It is virtually tasteless when the powder form is mixed with liquids (powder form is kosher). On the other hand, the ProFibe™ bar boasts a delicious satisfying taste in peanut butter, chocolate or cookie and cream and most importantly, contains 1½ servings of ProFibe powder. Also available is the Intro-Pack complete with one each of the three flavored meal replacement bars, a shaker cup, a 44 serving can of ProFibe and a new product – travel packets – 15 each in the flavor of classic orange and 15 each in strawberry kiwi.

For further information, visit www.profibe.com. To purchase by MasterCard or Visa, call 1-800-756-3999. Corporate Offices call 1-388-761-8100 fax to 1-366-761-2545.

Abbreviated Summary Recommendations

1. Cholesterol level recommendations.
2. American Heart Association tips for lower cholesterol.
3. Avoid high fructose corn syrup.
4. Eat fiber 30 to 35 grams
5. Nutrition and supplements that help lower cholesterol.
    a. Psyllum
    b. Policosanol
    c. Vitalzyme
    d. Omega-3 fatty acids
    e. Vitamin C
    f. Guggul
    g. Phytosterols
    h. ProFibe. This is a multi-prong supplement you will also find suggested to lower LDL in Chapter 13.

Note: This chapter or any other chapter in this book is not meant to dispense medical advice or strategies for your health care. It is meant to raise your awareness to be pro-active to other health options which should be discussed with your health care professional.

Chapter 12

Low HDL Spear

High-density lipoproteins [HDL]) form a class of lipoproteins, varying somewhat in their size [8-11 mm in diameter], that carry fatty acids and cholesterol from the body tissues to the liver. About thirty percent of blood cholesterol is carried by HDL.

The single biggest factor in the development of heart disease is determining the factor in the ratio of your total cholesterol to your HDL, e.g., cholesterol 150 ÷ by your HDL of 50 gives you a cholesterol HDL ratio of 3. The lower you can get below 4.2, the better. [Source: abstracted and edited: *Ultra Prevention*, authored by Mark Hyman and Mark Liponis, M.D.s.]

It is hypothesized that HDL can remove cholesterol from atheroma – *lipid deposits on lining of the artery* – within arteries and transport it back to the liver for excretion or re-utilization – which is the main reason why HDL-bound cholesterol is sometimes called "**good cholesterol**," or HDL. A high level of HDL-C seems to protect against cardiovascular disease and how HDL cholesterol levels [less than 40 mg/dL] increase the risk for heart disease. When measuring cholesterol, any contained in HDL particles is considered as protection to the body's cardiovascular health, in contrast to "bad" LDL cholesterol.

HDL particles are not inherently protective. It is only the HDL particles which become the largest [actually picking up and carrying cholesterol] which are protective. There is no reliable relationship between total HDL and large HDL, and more sophisticated analyses [VAP] which actually measure large HDL, not just total, correlate much better with clinical outcomes.

Historically, beginning in the late 1970s cholesterol and lipid assays were promoted to estimate total HDL-cholesterol because such tests used to be far less expensive, by about 50 fold, than measured lipoprotein particle concentrations and subclass analysis. Over time, with continued research, decreasing costs, greater availability and wider acceptance of other "lipoprotein subclass analysis" assay methods, including NMR spectroscopy, human studies have continued to show a stronger correlation between human clinically obvious cardiovascular events and quantitatively measured large HDL-particle concentrations.

Men tend to have noticeably lower HDL levels, with smaller size and lower cholesterol content, than women. Men also have an increased incidence of atherosclerotic heart disease [*No doubt due to the lower HDL level (author).*]

Epidemiology

Epidemiological studies have shown that high concentrations of HDL [over 60 mg/dL] have protective value against cardiovascular diseases such as ischemic stroke – *a blockage* – and myocardial infarction – *a blockage to the heart*. Low concentrations of HDL [below 40 mg/dL for men, below 50 mg/dL for women] are a positive risk factor for these atherosclerotic diseases.

Data from the landmark Framingham Heart Study showed that for a given low level of LDL, the risk of heart disease increases 10-fold as the DHL varies from high to low. Conversely, for a fixed low level of HDL, the risk increases 3-fold as LDL varies from low to high.

Even people with very low LDL levels are exposed to some increased risk if their HDL levels are not high enough. [Source: Philip Barker, M.D., "HDL Cholesterol, Very Low Levels of LDL Cholesterol, and Cardiovascular Events," *NEJM*, Sept. 27, 2007]

High HDL: Key to a Longer Life?

As people grow older, a high HDL level seems to be a good marker for longevity. Once someone reaches age 85, low levels of HDL cholesterol – rather than high levels of LDL cholesterol – are associated with an increased risk of death from heart disease and stroke, according to a recent Dutch study in the *Archives of Internal Medicine*.

In this study, a group of 599 individuals aged 85 years were followed for 4 years, during which time 152 of them died. People with low HDL levels were twice as likely to die of a heart attack and 2.5 more likely to have a fatal stroke, compared with those who had high HDL levels. Low HDL- as well as high LDL-levels more than doubled the risk of dying of infection.

Is it Genetic?

Research recently published in the *Journal of the American Medical Association* determined that many people who live exceptionally long, healthy lives – average age of study participants was 98 years – share a particular gene mutation that leads to higher HDL levels as well as larger HDL and LDL particles than those seen in the general population.

It has been suggested that large LDL particles may be protective against cardiovascular disease because such large particles cannot readily penetrate the walls of arteries and contribute to atherosclerosis. The gene mutation responsible for high HDL levels and bigger HDL and LDL particles appears to protect against many chronic diseases associated with aging, such as heart disease, stroke, and diabetes.

Although we are not all lucky enough to inherit the "longevity gene," there is much that we can do to raise our HDL level on our own – and perhaps increase our odds for a longer and healthier life.

[Source: *Johns Hopkins Medical Center*, "Health After 50," 6/05.]

Recommended Range

The American Heart Association, NIH and NCEP, provides a set of guidelines for male fasting HDL levels and risk for heart disease.

Level mg/dL	Interpretation
< 40	Low HDL cholesterol, heightened risk for heart disease, < 50 is the value for women.
40-59	Medium HDL level
> 60	High HDL level, optimal condition considered protective against heart disease

More sophisticated laboratory methods called VAP not only measure the total HDL but also the range of HDL particles, e.g., "lipoprotein subclass analysis," typically divided into several groups by size, instead of just the total HDL concentration as listed below. The largest groups [most functional] of HDL particles have the most protective effects. The groups of smallest particle reflect HDL particles which are not actively transporting cholesterol, thus not protective.

[Source abstracted and edited: Philip Barter, M.D., *NEJM*, Sept. 27, 2007.]

The pharmaceutical drug for raising your good cholesterol [HDL] never made it [thank the gods] to the market place.

This is another reason drugs should not be the first intervention of choice. Read on.

One of Pfizer's $800 million dollar nightmares is launching their new drug torcetrapib. It was withdrawn by Pfizer during this study. The drug torcetrapib had indeed lived up to expectations initially in that it did increase good cholesterol by 72% and reduced bad cholesterol by 24% in a study involving more than 15,000 patients. Although only 7,500 of the subjects received torcetrapib, all were administered atorvastatin, a powerful drug for lowering cholesterol that Pfizer sells under the brand name Lipitor. However, it was found in the study that in spite of this the chances of fatal heart problems climbed by 25% and deaths were up by 40%. Of the patients who took torcetrapib with Lipitor 93 died while 464 experienced "major cardiovascular events." The drug torcetrapib surprisingly also produced an unexpected "off-target" toxicity on the adrenal gland. This was instrumental in creating circumstances apt to damage artery walls and increase blood pressure.

[Source: abstracted and edited, Pfizer Pharmaceutical]

The pharmaceutical industry spends an average of 30 billion dollars per year on advertising. Of that $30 billion, $3.2 billion is spent on advertising directed at the consumer to consult their doctors about a particular medication. They also spend approximately $3,500 per physician to promote their drugs.

[Source: *Forbes Magazine*, 2005]

This has made Americans a prescription-dependent nation fascinated by the magical relief obtained in popping a pill.

It's a well-known medical fact that the good cholesterol HDL helps to protect you from a heart attack.

I have no way of knowing the cardiovascular profile of the volunteers in the study – *I am sure the quick fix of raising your HDL was the lure.*

I think I can say without fear of contradiction: In a perfect world, if Big Pharma didn't have a financial stranglehold on medical schools and the AMA did not spend 3.2 billion dollars on direct advertising to the consumer and did not spend approximately $3,500 on each physician to promote their drugs to their patients, we would turn to nutritional foods and supplements as our first interventions, and not prescription drugs. We then would all enjoy a healthier life.

Dr. Stephen Sinatra's recommendations for raising HDL:
- Niacin or as a prescription drug N-Aspan
- L Carnitine
- Co Q 10
- Pantethine

David W. Tanton, Ph.D.'s recommendations to raise HDL :
- Guggul – as stated in 7/2003 *Health Sense Nutritional Supplement*, published by the American Council on Collaborative Medicine, Inc. A study with 20 patients given guggul twice a day for 16 weeks raised HDL by 36%.
- Policosanol
- Curcumin. A small study indicated a 29% increase in HDL.
- Vitamin C.

Note: This chapter or any other chapter in this book is not meant to dispense medical advice or strategies for your health care. It is meant to raise your awareness to be pro-active to other health options which should be discussed with your health care professional.

CHAPTER 13

Elevated LDL Spear

What is Bad Cholesterol?

The medical term for "bad" cholesterol is low-density lipoprotein [LDL]. High levels of "bad" cholesterol in your body can clog your arteries and increase your risk of heart attack and stroke. That's the ugly truth. When there is too much bad cholesterol in your body, it can slowly build up in the walls of the arteries in your heart and brain. Once there, it can combine with other substances to form plaque, which can narrow your arteries and make them less flexible. This is a medical condition called atherosclerosis. If a blood clot forms and blocks an artery narrowed by plaque, you could have a heart attack or stroke. So for good health, keep you LDL low – below 100 mg/dL or lower, as advised by your health professional.

Dr. Stephen Sinatra, in his book *No More Heart Disease*, states:

"Your LDL reading is the best predictor of your risk of heart attack and stroke, with a higher score indicating a higher risk. LDL cholesterol levels can be broken into the following categories:

The American Heart Association, NIH and NCEP provide a set of guidelines for lowering LDL-Cholesterol levels, estimated or measured, and risk for heart disease. As of 2003, these guidelines were:

Level mg/dL	Level mmol/L	
< 100	< 2.6	Optimal LDL cholesterol, corresponding to reduced, but not zero, risk for heart disease
100 to 129	2.6 to 3.3	Near optimal LDL level
130 to 169	3.3 to 4.1	Borderline high LDL level
160 to 189	4.1 to 4.9	High LDL level
> 190	> 4.9	Very high LDL level, corresponding to highest increased risk of heart disease

These guidelines were based on a goal of presumably decreasing death rates from cardiovascular disease to less than 2 to 3%/year or less than 20 to 30%/10 years. Note that 100 is not considered optimal; less than 100 is optimal, though it is unspecified how much less.

Source: Wikipedia

Increasing evidence has revealed that the concentration and size of the LDL particles more powerfully relates to the degree of atherosclerosis progression than the concentration of cholesterol contained within all the LDL particles. The healthiest pattern, though relatively rare, is to have small numbers of large LDL particles and no small particles. Having small LDL particles, though common, is an unhealthy pattern; high concentrations of small LDL particles [even though potentially carrying the same total cholesterol content as a low concentration of large particles] correlates with much faster growth of atheroma – *progression of atherosclerosis* – and earlier and more severe cardiovascular disease events and death.

A complex set of biochemical reactions regulates the oxidation [*a chemical process degrading <u>radicals</u>*] as discussed – *in Chapter 8, Antioxidants and Free Radicals* – in the endothelium [*the inner lining of the artery*]. Nitric oxide down-regulates this oxidation process catalyzed by *L-Arginine*. The nutrient *L-Arginine* is a vital amino acid and is acknowledged for its antioxidant properties and is produced by your body. *I suggest you discuss with your health care professionals using an L-arginine supplement and its dosage.*

Dr. Roger H. Murphree states in his book, *Heart Disease: What Your Doctor Won't Tell You*: "LDL is not bad. It provides an essential bodily function. Only when LDL becomes oxidized from free radical proliferation does LDL become bad."

Can LDL be Too Low?

The medical community at Duke University in the late 1990s indicated with Low LDL levels [they did not give a precise number – *it was in the 70 to 80 mg range*] individuals suffered from various degrees of depression. There is also a speculation which indicates low LDL levels affected the way the cells receive serotonins to the brain, which causes depression.

My search to date indicates Harvard Medical School as well as the renowned Cleveland Heart Clinic recommend that anyone with heart disease get their LDL level down to 70.

Importance of Antioxidants

Dr. Sinatra further states in his book:

"Because LDL appears to be harmless until oxidized by free radicals, it is postulated that ingesting antioxidants and minimizing free radical exposure may reduce LDL's contribution to atherosclerosis, though results are not conclusive."

• L-arginine is an excellent antioxidant against free radicals as well as producing nitric acids to your blood.

<u>Note</u>: *Some supplements listed here you will find listed elsewhere as they have multi-prong benefits for other risk factors.*

Dr. Stephen Sinatra recommends:
1. Pantethine
2. Vit-E full spectrum alpha gamma and mixed tocepherols. They will also help prevent the oxidation of LDL as will tocotrienols, lutein, lycopene and green tea extract.

<u>Red Yeast Rice</u>:

In addition to its culinary use, red yeast rice is also used in traditional Chinese herbology and traditional Chinese medicine. Its use has been documented as far back as the Tang Dynasty in China in 800 A.D. and taken internally to invigorate the body, aid in digestion, and remove "blood blockages."

It is sold as an over-the-counter dietary supplement for controlling cholesterol. There is strong scientific evidence for its effect in lowering blood levels of total cholesterol, low-density lipoprotein/LDL ["bad" cholesterol], and triglyceride levels. Because an approved drug is identical to the molecule it is therefore regulated as a drug by the Food and Drug Administration [FDA]. *Red rice is a naturally occurring statin and therefore came under FDA jurisdiction.*

Herbs that are helpful to lower LDL:
1. Guggulipid – has performed better than modern drugs in many trials.
2. Turmeric – also helps blood circulation.
3. Green tea.

Additional helpers to lower LDL:
1. Chromium polyniconate
2. Psyllium husk - studies have shown psyllium husk effective in lowering LDL. Metamucil makes a wafer [*which is an excellent product*] containing psyllium. Each package contains two wafers which contain 6 grams of fiber.
3. Polycosanol – The Cleveland Clinic Men's Health Letter advisor 6/06 abstracted article about policosanol: "A 2002 review of 60 clinical trials concluded that policosanol lowered total cholesterol by 17 to 21 percent and LDL cholesterol by 21 to 29 percent, and raised HDL cholesterol by 8 to 15 percent. However, most research on policosanol comes from Cuba, and whether American-made policosanol products will have the same effects requires further study.
4. ProFibe [*abstracted from ProFibe literature*] – The medical community has been aware of the ability of water soluble dietary fibers [WSF] to naturally lower blood cholesterol LDL levels in humans.
   • Developed at the University of Florida by Dr. James Cerda and Charles Burgin, ProFibe is a patented, award-winning formula consisting of guar gum and citrus pectin complexed to non-GMOs [genetically modified] by protein. The result? A water soluble fiber supplement which is 100% usable by the body.

Usable water soluble fiber [WSF] can dramatically reduce cholesterol [LDL-C] levels by as much as 25-30% in one month! Other benefits may include reduced atherosclerosis, better digestion, improved glucose tolerance, weight loss and lowered blood pressure. Many ProFibe users report enhanced energy levels as well.

• **Case Study I**
   A 58 year-old white male taking 10 mg of Zocor one/day. His total cholesterol was 221. His LDL-C was 137 and his triglycerides were 243. ProFibe was introduced at three servings per day with the 10 mg of Zocor, for 30 days. At the end of the 30 days the subject's total cholesterol was 159, LDL-C was 86 and the triglycerides were 187. The risk factor improved from 3.9 to 2.4.

- **Case Study II**

A 53 year-old white female taking 10 mg of Zocor per day. Her total cholesterol of 249, her LDL-C was 158 and her triglycerides were 198. At the end of 30 days of taking three servings per day of ProFibe with the 10 mg of Zocor, the total cholesterol was 216, LDL-C was 134 and triglycerides were 130. Risk factor improved from 3.1 to 2.4.

- **Case Study III**

A 61 year-old white female with a recent history of CAD. Taking 20 mg per day of Mevacor, she had a total cholesterol of 301, and an LDL-C of 141. After taking three servings per day of ProFibe with the Mevacor for only 14 days, the total cholesterol dropped to 217 and the LDL-C fell to 84. The risk factor dropped from 4.7 to 3.2.

Not only is ProFibe™ safe and proven effective, it is easy to use. Three servings a day are recommended, which supplies a whopping 18 mg of fiber, over one-half of the daily recommended amount. This provides as much beneficial WSF [water-soluble fiber] as a bucket of oatmeal, a dozen oranges or a bushel of apples! Yet you cannot receive the same healthy benefits from fruit alone or other supplements on the market. It is virtually tasteless when the powder form is mixed with liquids [powder form is kosher]. On the other hand, the ProFibe™ bar boasts a delicious satisfying taste in peanut butter, chocolate or cookie and cream and most importantly, contains 1½ servings of ProFibe powder. Also available is the Intro-Pack complete with one each of the three flavored meal replacement bars, a shaker cup, a 44 serving can of ProFibe and a new product – travel packets – 15 each in the flavor of classic orange and 15 each in strawberry kiwi.

For further information, visit www.profibe.com. To purchase by MasterCard or Visa, call 1-800-756-3999. Corporate Offices call 1-388-761-8100 fax to 1-366-761-2545.

Note: This chapter or any other chapter in this book is not meant to dispense medical advice or strategies for your health care. It is meant to raise your awareness to be pro-active to other health options which should be discussed with your health care professional.

Chapter 14

Elevated Triglycerides Spear

Triglycerides: A Big Fat Problem

This forgotten fat is a source of confusion – and heart disease.

Why is it that the most common form of fat in food and in the bloodstream is the one that's most often ignored? <u>Triglycerides take a backseat to low-density lipoprotein [LDL] and high density lipoprotein [HDL] largely because their precise role in heart disease has been something of a mystery.</u>

That's changing. Researchers are getting a grip on how triglycerides add to atherosclerosis, the artery-clogging process which is the root of most heart disease. This knowledge may change how triglycerides are measured and when they need to be treated.

<u>The Trouble with Triglycerides</u>

Good fats, bad fats, and in-between fats have one thing in common: they all contain triglycerides. These particles consist of three fatty acid chains linked by an alcohol called glycerol. When you eat a cheeseburger, your digestive system rips apart the triglycerides [the fat] in the meat and cheese into their individual fatty acids. These are small enough to enter intestinal cells called enterocytes. Enterocytes stitch together fatty acids into new triglycerides, pack them with protein and cholesterol into huge particles called chylomicrons, and release them into the bloodstream. Chylomicrons ferry triglycerides to tissues, where they are burned for energy or stored. <u>The liver also packages triglycerides into large particles called very-low-density lipoproteins [VLDs].</u>

As chylomicrons and VLDs give up their fats to the body's cells, they shrink, becoming dense, cholesterol-rich particles. One of these is LDL, which readily burrows into artery walls. This is a key early step in the process that ends with cholesterol buildup in arteries.

<u>Transformation into LDL isn't the only issue with high blood levels of triglycerides. The more abundant they are, the less HDL the body makes. That's a problem, because HDL scavenges LDL from the blood and from artery walls.</u>

<u>Measuring Up</u>

The amount of triglycerides in the bloodstream rises and falls throughout the day. After a fatty meal, triglycerides can be so abundant they give blood a milky tint. Within a few hours, they're mostly cleared out. Doctors traditionally test for triglycerides after an overnight fast so the results aren't thrown off by what you've just eaten. Categories are based on these fasting levels [see "Triglyceride Levels"].

Two recent reports in the *Journal of the American Medical Association* suggested that testing for triglycerides two to four hours after a meal offers a better gauge of their impact on heart disease.

One study followed almost 14,000 Danes for more than 25 years. Women with the highest nonfasting triglyceride levels at the start of the study were five times more likely to have died from a heart attack or other cardiac event than women with the lowest levels. <u>For men, high triglycerides doubled the risk</u>. The second study, conducted by Harvard researchers, followed 26,000 women for more than 10 years. Triglyceride levels measured two to four hours after eating – but not fasting triglyceride levels – were linked with heart attacks and other cardiovascular problems.

It's possible that people who don't clear triglycerides quickly are exposed to their dense, atherosclerosis-causing byproducts for longer than people who get rid of them quickly. It's also possible that triglycerides lingering in the bloodstream is a signal that muscle and other tissues are becoming resistant to insulin.

<u>Triglyceride Boosters</u>

Fatty foods aren't the only cause of high blood levels of triglycerides. Other contributors include :
- eating a lot of rapidly digested carbohydrates
- an underactive thyroid gland
- kidney disease
- diabetes
- overproduction of the hormones aldosterone or cortisol
- excess weight, especially extra pounds around the waist
- inactivity
- smoking
- medications such as high-dose thiazide diuretics or beta blockers, estrogen, tamoxifen, steroids, isotretionin, and some anti-HIV drugs.

Inheritance also plays a role. Some people have high triglycerides due to genetic disorders, such as familial combined hyperlipidemia and familial hypertriglyceridemia.
<u>Very High Triglycerides</u>

When fasting triglycerides shoot above 500 mg/dL, more than the heart and arteries may be at risk. <u>Pancreatitis is often seen with triglyceride levels above 1,000 mg/dL</u>. Near 2,000 mg/dL they can trigger a harmful buildup of fat in the liver and retina. They can also spark the eruption of itchy, pimple-like xanthomas [zen-THOE-mus] on the hands, feet, arms, legs, and buttocks.

If you are diagnosed with very high triglycerides, a search for causes related to genes, disease, or medication is in order. Controlling such high levels usually includes a very low-fat diet [under 15% of calories from fat], no alcohol, and triglyceride-lowering nutritional supplements and if required, prescription drugs.

What's the Risk?

One reason triglycerides have long been shunted into the background is that their precise connection with heart disease has been iffy – some studies have shown a connection, others haven't. The latest meta-analysis, published last year in *Circulation*, combined the results of 29 studies with more than 260,000 participants. In this report, people with high triglyceride levels were 70% more likely to have developed heart disease over an average of 10 years than those with normal levels. Some of this increase disappeared, though, when high LDL, low HDL, and other cardiac risk factors were taken into account.

At first glance, the statement ["Some of this increase disappeared, though when high LDL, low HDL, and other cardiac risk factors were taken into account"] might seem confusing. What they simply mean is, if they had removed the risk factors of high LDL, low HDL and other cardiac risk factors, it would have lowered the high triglyceride effect.

That disappearance captures the big controversy over triglycerides; Are they harmful on their own, or are they stand-ins for other problems? It's a difficult question to answer, since high triglycerides are usually part of a pack of problems that also includes low HDL, high blood pressure, high blood sugar, and a large waist. These run together; they are called metabolic syndrome.

In other people, high triglycerides are a lone wolf. Even when they stand alone, however, they predispose individuals to heart disease.

High Triglycerides May Increase Stroke Risk

The 12/26/07 issue of *Neurology* reported: Researches examining the 4-year records of 1,049 patients admitted to hospitals who had a stroke or transient ischemic attack mini-stroke]. Among them, 247 had an atherosclerotic stroke which is a type of stroke caused by a blockage in the large arteries supplying blood to the brain. Those with the highest triglyceride levels were about 2.7 times more likely to suffer this type of stroke than those with the lowest levels.

Source: abstracted and edited, *Cleveland Clinic Men's Health Advisor*, 3/08.

Targeting Triglycerides

When high triglycerides are accompanied by high LDL and low HDL – the usual scenario – they aren't the main focus of therapy. Guidelines recommend going after high LDL first, usually with a statin drug. *Nutritional supplements should be your first choice of intervention.* Then it's time to work on triglycerides and HDL. Unless your triglycerides are extremely high, lifestyle changes are the best place to start. These can lead to impressive reductions in triglycerides.

Beware of bad fats. Cutting back on saturated fat [in red meat and dairy foods] and trans fats [in restaurant fried food and commercially prepared baked goods] can lower triglycerides.

Go for good carbs. <u>Easily digested carbohydrates [white bread, white rice, cornflakes, and sugared soda] raise triglyceride levels</u>. Eating whole grains and cutting back on sugared soda can help control triglycerides.

Check your alcohol. Moderate drinking is good for the heart. But in some people, alcohol dramatically boosts triglycerides. The only way to know if you are one of these "responders" is to avoid alcohol for a few weeks and have your triglycerides tested again.

Go fish. Omega-3 fats in salmon, tuna, sardines, and other fatty fish can lower triglycerides. Having fish twice a week is fine.

Aim for healthy weight. If you are overweight, losing 5% to 10% of your weight can help drive down triglycerides. Losing more is even better.

Get moving. Exercise lowers triglycerides and boosts HDL.

Stop smoking. It isn't good for triglyceride levels or anything else.

<u>Not to be ignored</u>

The body needs some triglycerides in order to function properly. Too much of them can tip you toward heart disease or make it worse. Finding a balance can be tricky.

Some doctors turn a blind eye to triglycerides unless they are really, really high. That's not such a good idea. If your triglycerides are in the danger zone, above 200 mg/dL, try to bring them down by changing your diet, using nutritional supplements, getting more exercise, and taking a triglyceride-lowering medication if needed. The payoff of these remedies is a healthier heart.

Triglyceride Levels	
Classification:	- ranges
Normal	- Less than 150
Borderline	- 150-199
High	- 200-499
Very high	- 500 or higher

*Values in milligrams per deciliter [mg/dL].

Source: National Cholesterol Education Program.

<u>Suggested Natural Interventions for Elevated Triglycerides</u>

The 2003 European Prospective Investigation into Cancer and Nutrition, which spanned 10 countries and included 519,978 participants who were observed for nearly five years, found that those with the highest amounts of fiber in their diets had a 40% lower risk of developing colon cancer than those with the lowest fiber intake. Other recent studies have found that increasing daily fiber intake by 10 grams lowers the risk of all coronary events by 14% and reduces the risk of death from heart disease by 27%. <u>Fiber has been found to lower levels of triglycerides</u>, low-density lipoprotein [LDL], C-reactive protein, and blood pressure – all of which are independent risk factors for heart attack and stroke.

Source: Dr. Steven A. Schnur, founder of South Florida Cardiology Associates, largest cardiology practice in South Florida; author of Reality Diet.

The more we know about fish oils . . .the closer we come to eliminate diseases of the cardiovascular system.

As the editor writes in *The American Journal of Cardiology*

"There has been considerable research into the effects of omega-3 fatty acids on cardiovascular disease since the initial studies of Greenland Eskimos 30 years ago. While we now use omega-3 fatty acids as a therapeutic approach to managing dyslipodemia and reducing cardiovascular risk, there remain many unanswered questions about the mechanism of action of this treatment and the magnitude of the cardiovascular event reduction benefit we can expect."

Overall, the benefits of fish oils for reducing the risk by 50% or more of heart and vascular disease, or heart attack, of sudden cardiac death, or stroke, have been established by dozens of studies in the past 30 years. That is, for example: The Physicians Health Study, which compared morbidity and survival rates of 20,000 men, some of whom consumed no fish, others who consumed fish at least once weekly; the Nurses Health Study that used food frequency diaries to assess dietary intake of omega-3 fatty acids and fish consumption over a 10-year period; the Cardiovascular Health Study involving 4775 over 12 years. Because results have been positive, <u>these studies and others like them of fish oils benefits are certain to be ongoing and very effective in lowering elevated triglycerides.</u>

• ***Guggul.*** Documentation shows that **the herb known as guggul outperforms prescription pharmaceuticals in the reduction of total cholesterol, <u>lowering triglycerides</u> and increasing the HDL level**. As stated in the July 2003 *Health Sense Nutritional Supplement*, published by The American Council on Collaborative Medicine, Inc. [ACCM], in one study, 20 patients with high cholesterol were given guggul two times a day for 16 weeks, resulting in cholesterol levels that dropped 22%, <u>triglycerides down 27%</u> and HDL up by 36%. Another study showed it reduced the tendency of blood to clot by 30%.

• ***Garlic*** lowers cholesterol, <u>triglycerides levels</u>, and blood pressure, as well as protecting against cardiovascular disease, available in tasteless and odorless forms. For best results, take 2 capsules, 3 times daily.

• ***Sugar*** can produce a significant rise in triglycerides, such as processed fruit juices.

• Food containing ***hydrogenated or partially hydrogenated oils*** [which become transfatty acids in the blood stream], such as most crackers, chips, cakes, candies, cookies [yes, and Girl

Scout cookies, too], margarine, doughnuts, peanut butter, processed cheese, and so on can substantially raise triglycerides.

• *Limit your daily fat intake* to 20% [5% max. of which is saturated fat] of your total calorie intake.

• *Carnitine* lowers blood triglyceride levels.
Source: Abstracted and edited, David W. Tanton, Ph.D., author of *Drug Free Approach to Health Care.*

Note: This chapter or any other chapter in this book is not meant to dispense medical advice or strategies for your health care. It is meant to raise your awareness to be pro-active to other health options which should be discussed with your health care professional.

CHAPTER 15

C-Reactive Protein [CRP]

My research has revealed controversy between some of the rock stars of the medical community.

The controversy is over a microscopic protein [C-Reactive Protein] which may be a prophetic predictor of heart disease and be the missing link as to whether a high blood level of CRP increases your risk of heart attack or a stroke.

The protein, which can be detected in a blood test, is a signal that inflammation is flaring somewhere in the body. And the discovery is believed by many experts – ranging from those at the American Heart Association to others at the U.S. Center for Disease Control and Prevention – to confirm the theory that inflammatory processes are involved in cardiovascular disease.

Indeed, the heart association, CDC and the American College of Cardiology had gone on record two years ago endorsing routine testing to determine CRP levels. Experts at all three organizations say screening is one way to identify cardiac patients who otherwise would not be found.

Elevated CRP levels, these experts say, may explain cases of heart disease that can't be blamed on high levels of low density lipoprotein, LDL, the so-called bad form of cholesterol, the key component in artery-clogging plaque.

Some prefer to wait and see

Despite the hoopla, many top heart specialists say they are taking a wait-and-see approach. For now, they're not ordering the test because the findings came from research limited to patients who had been treated for previous cardiovascular disease. What hasn't been established, they say, is whether CRP is a risk factor for those without known cardiovascular problems.

Once believed to be an innocent bystander in the debris that makes up plaque, CRP now is considered, at least by some doctors, nearly as potent a culprit in heart disease as the bad form of cholesterol. It is produced in cells that line vessel walls and in the liver. The protein flows into the bloodstream when inflammation flares anywhere in the body.

Inflammation is the body's response to injury or irritation and is characterized by the army of warrior cells and proteins that pour from the immune system to defend the injured site. Inflammation, with its tendency to produce heat and swelling, can cause injury. In the case of blood vessels, inflammatory processes can damage vascular walls, and thus is another path to atherosclerosis, doctors say.

Dr. Stacey Rosen, chief of cardiology at Long Island-Jewish Medical Center in New Hyde Park, N/Y/ hasn't yet turned to routine CRP testing.

"I think the correlation [documented in the study] is fascinating," she said, adding that because the studies involved only people who had coronary artery disease, the jury is still out.

Dr. Thomas Nicosia, director of cardiology at St. Francis Hospital, The Heart Center in Roslyn, N.Y. also wants to see more scientific work on the protein. "Right now, it's one of the players in the mix of components that make up plaque in blood vessels," Nicosia said.

And there is more skepticism.

"I don't think we're yet at the point where routine measurement of CRP is warranted," said Dr. Robert Phillips, a cardiologist and chairman of medicine at Lenox Hill Hospital in Manhattan, N.Y. "We have not yet teased out whether CRP is completely independent from LDL as a cause of atherosclerosis," the artery-damaging disorder caused by plaque.

Even these physicians believe that inflammation plays an active role in cardiovascular disease. The open question is whether the recent research is the confirmation most cardiologists had been awaiting.

Dr. Robert Phillips of Lenox Hill Hospital in New York remains steadfast in not jumping on the CRP bandwagon.

While inflammation is an important aspect of cardiovascular disease, he said he prefers to prescribe aspirin, the old medicine cabinet standby for inflammation.

Many questions remain for Dr. Harvey Hecht, director of preventive cardiology at Beth Israel Medical Center in Manhattan, N.Y., who said many matters regarding CRP remain unanswered. It will take time before doctors discern whether screening has widespread benefit.

"I think two things need to happen in order to use CRP to [routinely] screen patients," he said. "You need convincing evidence to add to our existing measures, and right now that data is lacking. You also need to show that lowering CRP is warranted."

CPR could rival LDL as cause

Still, inflammation is so prevalent in damaged arteries, some researchers say, that the CRP link to cardiovascular risk could rival the cholesterol hypothesis that has stood firm for more than half a century: that LDL cholesterol is the underlying cause of heart attacks and strokes.

Doctors who strongly endorse CRP's role as a player nearly equal to LDL believe it could prove to be the missing link that explain why some people who lack a genetic predisposition to heart disease and who have normal cholesterol, blood glucose, blood pressure and weight go on to have heart attacks and strokes.

But CRP is "a big part of the explanation," said Dr. Paul Ridker, pioneering heart researcher at Brigham and Women's Hospital in Boston and the lead author of one of the two studies, published in January in the *New England Journal of Medicine.* "Half of all heart attacks occur in people with perfectly normal cholesterol levels," added Ridker, who directs the hospital's Center for Cardiovascular Disease Prevention and co-developed the test universally used to detect CRP. Brigham and Women's Hospital holds the patent. Both studies received funding from pharmaceutical companies.

Several smaller studies since the 1990s of healthy people and those with heart disease have demonstrated that when CRP levels are high, the risk for heart attacks and strokes increases.

"We had already published overwhelming evidence showing that people with high CRP and high LDL are at very high risk," Ridker said. His latest work bolsters those findings and shows that cholesterol-lowering statin drugs can also lower levels of CRP.

Ridker and other proponents of testing say it is as important for people to know their CRP level as to know their cholesterol levels. He and other doctors who favor screening underscore the test's simplicity. It's one of those preventive measures, they say, that can't hurt – and might help.

CRP testing is not for everyone. People with any rheumatoid condition, such as arthritis or lupus, or chronic infections would not be ideal candidates because their levels of CRP are high, a result of the generalized inflammation associated with their disorders.

The American Heart Association reports that an average CRP reading of 1 or lower is desirable. At levels of 3 and above, the risk for heart attack and stroke rises substantially. The CDC backs the test because an estimated 40 percent of U.S. adults are at risk of heart disease.

Inflammation relationship

Many doctors say it is critical to detect inflammation because of its role in a number of disease processes. In addition to cardiovascular damage, scientists increasingly are pointing to inflammation as an underlying cause of cancer, Alzheimer's disease and autoimmune disorders, in which the body attacks itself. CRP signals inflammation's role in damage to the heart, Ridker and other doctors say.

"The evidence is very, very strong," said Dr. Steven Nissen, vice chairman of cardiology at the Cleveland Clinic and lead investigator of the second study. Both analyses found that CRP points to elevated inflammation in the arteries and that cholesterol-lowering statin drugs can diminish levels of the protein.

The two research projects have paved the way for potentially hundreds of thousands of new patients to take cholesterol-lowering medications such as Lipitor, Crestor, Mevacor, Zocor and Pravacol.

Source: abstracted and edited, *Newsday*, 3/1/2005.

While these medical rock stars argue over the risk status consideration of CRP, my suggestion is that you should include having your blood tested for it when they do a lipid profile evaluation.

High Sensitivity CRP (HSCRP) ranges
< 1.0   LOW
1.0 – 3.0   AVERAGE
> 3.0   HIGH

I would certainly expect that Dr. Ridker, who holds the patent for the CRP test, which, if you noticed, that the study was funded by the pharmaceutical companies and Dr. Steven Nissen, chairman of cardiology at the Cleveland Clinic, both traditional medicine doctors recommend statins for lowering CRP *and not nutritional supplements.*

Recommendations for non-statins for lowering CRP:

- if you haven't done so yet, stop smoking
- exercise
- lose weight
- take CoQ10, omega-3 fish oils, vitamin E
- take Gingko Biloba [don't combine with aspirin as it accelerates bleeding]
- garlic and ginger are other nutrients that help combat inflammation and clotting characteristics of CRP.

Life Extension Foundation recommendations for lowering CRP:
- eat low glycemic index foods
- reduce intake of omega-6 fatty acids
- take DHEA [dehydroepiandrosterone], it is currently a prescription drug.
- take vitamin C
- CRP seems to reduce levels of A, C. E, carotenoids, zinc and selenium. You should emphasize taking these nutrients for your overall cardio health.

Note: This chapter or any other chapter in this book is not meant to dispense medical advice or strategies for your health care. It is meant to raise your awareness to be pro-active to other health options which should be discussed with your health care professional.

CHAPTER 16

Elevated Homocysteine Spear

What is Homocysteine? The amino acid that gets no respect from the AHA & AMA.

"Homocysteine is a byproduct of the conversion of the amino acid into methionine. If homocysteine is not converted into methionine, it will become oxidized by free radicals. It then starts to accumulate in the endothelia [lining] cells of the arterial wall. This leads to plaque formation and possible arterial occlusion. Homocysteine speeds up the oxidation [causing toxic damage] of cholesterol, which then becomes bound to small LDL particles. Macrophages [white blood cells] then infiltrate the particles and transform them into plaque. This plaque begins to grow within the arterial lining. Cholesterol swimming through the blood stream attempts to patch the damaged arterial lining and more plaque occurs."

Source: Dr. Rodger Murphree, author of *Heart Disease: What Your Doctor Won't Tell You.*

"Dr. Kilmer McCulley first suggested almost 40 years ago that elevated levels of homocysteine were associated with an increased risk of CAD [carotid artery disease]. He based his theories on autopsies he and other pathologists conducted on children with a genetic disease called homocysteinuria who has also had advanced coronary artery disease. Dr. McCulley was brazen enough to suggest that cholesterol wasn't promoting arteriosclerosis; the toxic byproduct known as homocysteine was.

A major cover-up occurred as he was pressured not to publish his findings due to the tremendous profit potential of the statin [cholesterol lowering] drugs. He persisted and published his findings, which cost him his job at Harvard Medical School and his funding. Unfortunately, the information was not acted upon, but was instead suppressed and the statin drugs, which have no effect on homocysteine, are still being aggressively marketed today.

This is a prime example of what Dr. Paul Rosch, M.D. was referring to at a conference held in 2003 in Arlington, Virginia, when he indicated that half of all heart attacks occur in people with normal cholesterol levels, and stressed that" *Anyone who questions cholesterol usually finds his funding cut off"* [http://www.medicalconsumers.org/page/cholesterol skeptics.html]. Fortunately, I am funding my own research."

Curiosity doesn't always kill that cat.

After writing chapter two and researching Big Pharmas' manipulation of medical schools and the AMA, the following isolated facts seem to have a common thread with Dr. McCulley.

My research found:

- Statin drugs hit the market approximately 17 years ago in 1990.
- According to the *Journal of Health Affairs*, as reported by Bloomberg/*Philadelphia Inquirer*, it takes average drugs tested 10 years before they hit the market.
- Therefore, it would put statin drug testing starting well before 1980. *This means this drug was in the pipeline earlier than 1980 during the same period Dr. McCulley was working on his book.*
- Dr. Kilmer McCulley's book, *The Homocysteine Revolution*, published by Keats Publishing in 1979.
- He probably worked on the book for at least several years while he was at Harvard. *That means it must have been common knowledge at Harvard that Dr. McCulley was going to publish a book on homocysteine.*
- Total revenues in 2007 for statin drugs exceeded 22 billion dollars. You don't have to have a spoon-bending mind to feel this is more than a coincidence that Big Pharma's fingerprints were all over Harvard's severance package [ask to resign] to Dr. McCulley for his great medical achievement.

Numerous studies now available validate Dr. McCulley's theory. The *European Journal of Medicine* reported that 40% of those who had strokes also had elevated homocysteine levels.

Framingham Heart Study: A Leading Researcher

"Cardiovascular disease [CVD] is the leading cause of death and serious illness in the United States. In 1948, the Framingham Heart Study – under the direction of the National Heart Institute [now known as the National Heart, Lung, and Blood Institute: NHLB] – embarked on an ambitious project in health research. At the time, little was known about the general causes of heart disease and stroke, but the death rates for CVD had been increasing steadily since the beginning of the century and had become an American epidemic.

The Objective of the Framingham Heart Study was to identify the common factors or characteristics that contribute to CVD by following its development over a long period of time in a large group of participants who had not yet developed overt symptoms of CVD or suffered a heart attack or stroke.

The researchers recruited 5,209 men and women between the ages of 30 and 62 from the town of Framingham, Massachusetts, and began the first round of extensive physical examinations and lifestyle interviews that they would later analyze for common patterns related to CVD development."

1986. First report on dementia was published revealing that autopsies of people that had died from Alzheimer's disease indicated that their homocysteine levels exceeded 13.5 umoL/L.

1990. Their study indicated homocysteine [an amino acid] was found to be a possible risk factor for heart disease.

"A Norwegian study involving over 4,700 men and women showed that each 5-millimol/L increase in homocysteine blood plasma caused the number of deaths from all sources to jump to 40%. This included a 50% increase in cardiovascular deaths and a 26% increase in cancer deaths.

- Homocysteine and cognitive function in elderly people [CMAJ 2004 Oct. 12:171[8]:897-904].

There is evidence that increased serum homocysteine levels are associated with declining cognitive function and dementia.

- Effect of homocysteine-lowering therapy with folic acid, vitamin B-12, and vitamin B-6 on clinical outcome after percutaneous [internal] coronary interventions: The Swiss Heart Study: a randomized controlled trial [JAMA 2002 Aug. 28:288[8]:973-9].

Conclusion: Homocysteine-lowering with folic acid, vitamin B-12 and vitamin B-6 may significantly decreases the incidence of major adverse cardio events after percutaneous [internal] coronary interventions.

Based on random hospital blood tests, the prevalence of elevated homocysteine in the elderly with chronic illnesses is estimated to be at 60 to 70%. Seventy percent of those with vascular disease had elevated homocysteine levels, and 63% of those with cognitive dysfunction had elevated homocysteine levels.

High homocysteine levels can be caused by foods – red meat, avocados, sunflower seeds, wild game, poultry, and ricotta cheese. These foods contain the amino acid methionine. If you don't get enough B vitamins, your body cannot break down methionine, resulting in homocysteine.

These deficiencies can be further exacerbated by caffeine and alcohol, which cause excessive urination and wash out precious B vitamins from our bodies.

Research also shows that five percent of the population may have inherited a rare genetic enzymatic defect that leads to higher homocysteine levels and premature heart disease. Because of this genetic data, the evaluation of serum homocysteine levels should become standard in preventive cardiology, especially in anyone with a family history of premature heart disease.

There is plenty of interest today in homocysteine, as evidenced by the abundance of information available in the medical and nutrition literature, as well as on the Internet; because elevated homocysteine has been linked to just about every ailment you can think of: heart attack, stroke, peripheral vascular disease, diabetes, obesity, dementia, Alzheimer's disease, osteoporosis, and pregnancy complications. Numerous studies have been conducted in recent times to confirm these links. <u>Is it any wonder that serious health-minded persons are committed to monitoring and controlling their homocysteine level</u>?

Elevated homocysteine levels can contribute to heart disease in at least three ways: (1) a direct toxic effect that damages the cells' lining on the inside of the coronary arteries; (2) contributing to arterial blood clotting [thrombosis]; and (3) facilitating the bad effects of LDL cholesterol."

However, conventional medicine does not react to these studies and, therefore, there is much controversy regarding physicians even considering and in most cases not including homocysteine testing when they order a Lipid or VAP profile performed on their patients.

This posture by the AMA and AHA is also indicated by the non-AMA & AHA regulated standards that the labs use in reporting homocysteine levels. *A national survey in 2006 published in the New England Journal of Medicine in which 94 percent of the doctors polled said they had "direct ties" with the drug industry. Do you think they have any interest with homocysteine as a serious risk factor?*

These ranges are [for the most part] with few exceptions 5 to 15 umoL/L.

In spite of these ranges, some of my research indicates the following:

- Dr. Stephen Sinatra recommends levels above 9 to be dangerous.
- Dr. Frederick Vagnini states, 10 or above are above normal and are dangerous [although, opinions differ on the number] homocysteine levels.
- Life Extension Foundation recommends people keep their homocysteine levels between 7 to 9. A homocysteine level over 12 should be treated very aggressively.
- Mark Hyman and Mark Liponis, M.D.s, medical doctors of the Canyon Ranch in the Berkshires, Massachusetts recommend a homocysteine less than 9.
- Dr. Rodger H. Murphree, author of *Heart Disease: What Your Doctor Won't Tell You*, recommends homocysteine levels should be kept under 6.3. He further states laboratories generally advocate that homocysteine levels are normal up to 15.

"Lately [2006] – the American Heart Association and the major medical journals have recognized the importance of folic acid and vitamins B6 and B12 for lowering homocysteine levels in the blood as a defense against cardiovascular problems. In one reported study, researchers found a direct measurable relationship between blood homocysteine levels and the severity of the atherosclerosis."

Even at this point in time the American Heart Association does not publish recommended homocysteine ranges because it seems to consider it a risk factor but not a serious risk factor.

This particular homocysteine spear strikes me very personally for the following reasons:

My very good friend [or so I thought, he and his family enjoyed ski weekends at our condo at Stratton, VT on many weekends and, of more significant importance, my wife and I were married at his North Shore Estate on Long Island], you remember, that was the internist I was seeing for 20 years. I asked him for a homocysteine evaluation – *I had read about in Dr. Sinatra's newsletter* – as you know, it came back 13.5.

I kept records on my lipo profile, 14 (of the 20 years) which I averaged out to:

cholesterol	222	certainly respectable – *but only 22 points over normal.*
HDL	55	> 35 is normal
LDL	143	that is 13 above high normal range
triglycerides	132	< 151 is normal.

Ratio HDL to cholesterol 4.2 [below 5 was considered a safe range; it's now 4.2].

I later found out when I became my own health advocate, I had moderate aortic valve stenosis and moderate to severe right interior carotid artery stenosis: both being asymptomatic.

My hypothesis based on the 14 year average lipid profile and my subsequent high homocysteine levels were the cause. Since my HDL to cholesterol level was in a safe range, the high homocysteine levels were the culprit.

My <u>very</u> ex-internist favorite "cutting edge" doctors speak was, "if it walks like a duck, looks like a duck, and sounds like a duck – it must be a duck."

Using his logic, it was the homocysteine.
Over the last 6 years since I left him, I have taken variations of:
B-12 – 1000 mcg
B-6 – 250 mg and a more bio-available form of B-6 P5P [predoxal 5 phosphate]
Folic acid ranges – 800 mcg to 3200 mcg.

Also using
TMG [trimethyglycine] up to 6000 mg

This only produced an average of 11.70 over the 6 years [not very good according to my research]. But according to the lab ranges very acceptable.

It seems since I did not respond to the generally recommended protocol to lower your homocysteine, I must be in the 5% of the population who have inherited a rare genetic enzymatic defect that leads to higher homocysteine levels and premature heart disease.

Homocysteine and Supplements

"While the AHA does not explicitly recommend supplements, it strongly advises patients at risk 'to be sure to get enough folic acid and vitamin B-6 and B-12 in their diet. They should eat fruits and green, leafy vegetables daily.' At the AHA's recommendation, the U.S. Food and Drug Administration has mandated that all <u>white flour</u> be 'enriched' with folic acid. National advisories are always on the conservative side so as to have broadest application. In clinical practice, however, many factors are taken into account in treating the individual patient: family history, the patient's diet, and other risk factors, such as smoking or obesity. The safest path to follow is to take advantage of every positive therapy available. That's true for supplements, especially since many persons do not get enough vitamins in their usual daily diets.

Health problems with homocysteine can arise in several ways: (1) genetic predisposal to a high homocysteine level; (2) a kinetic disorder in which homocysteine is not adequately flushed from the blood stream; (3) a poor dietary habit with lack of fruits and vegetables; (4) with obesity and diabetes; (5) lack of hydrochloric acid, which is produced by the parietal cells in the stomach. The parietal cells also produce an intrinsic factor which is required for absorption of B-12. In addition, hydrochloric acid is also required for absorption of folic acid.

In general, men have higher levels of homocysteine than women, most likely due to higher creatinine values and greater muscle mass. Women, before menopause, have lower levels of homocysteine than do postmenopausal women. Any one of the above conditions may be the cause of a high homocysteine level."

The standard B vitamins used to lower elevated homocysteine levels in people who do not have a rare genetic enzymatic defect are:

• Folic acid
• B-6
• B-12

There are variations and additions to the standard recommendations:

• B-12 – methyl cobalamin – sublingual, in place of regular B-12
• B-6 – pyridoxal 5 phosphate – in place of regular B-6
• Folinic acid
• Metafolin – in place of folic acid
• TMG [trimethylglycine, also called betaine]
• Riboflavin
• Garlic
• Omega-3

I was curious that the AHA did not set standards for homocysteine [at least my research did not find them], but set standards for the lipid profile [e.g., cholesterol, HDL, LDL, and triglycerides].

I could not come to grips with the disparity that the majority of physicians who I had researched – *which are integrated/complementary physicians* – who had an average high normal of under 9, and the lab's ranges which were being used of 5 to 15. I think the 5 to 15 range gives doctors, and therefore their patients, a false sense of a no-risk factor if a patient is over 9 or 10.

I remember the AHA years back had a 300 cholesterol as normal. Now it's 200.
The JNC up until 2003 had 130/80 as normal, now over 120/80 is prehypertensive.
But laboratories are using 5 to 15 range. Where did these range standards originate?

I called the Bio Reference Lab main office in Nassau County and spoke to Cathy Philip, the Q & A Manager. I asked her who set the 5 to 15 range on homocysteine that their lab used. Cathy told me the manufacturer of the chemicals and instruments that Bio Reference used in calculating the homocysteine levels in their lab. When I asked Cathy where the manufacturer got the ranges from, Cathy was told from a General Population Study.

Cathy said Bio Reference would then do an essay study among 50 to 100 of the patients and tweak the manufacturer ranges.

In my view, this defies logic. Why the AHA and AMA who have access to the largest data bases in probably the world, but still refuse to recognize the serious risk factor of homocysteine and will not set standards and ranges and have it included with all lipo profile work, have just earned my endorsement for the Rodney Dangerfield Award for homocysteine. "It gets no respect."

Ask yourself, if it's the manufacturer who was setting the homocysteine range for homocysteine from a "general population study" wouldn't it be a logical conclusion that the general population has very high ranges of homocysteine? *If this hypothesis is correct it's due to the complete indifference of the AHA & AMA toward homocysteine as a serious risk factor.*

If the AHA and the AMA had set standards as they did with lipid profiles and the [JNC7] had with blood pressure and had collected the overwhelming data that lowered cholesterol from a normal 300 to its present 200 and [JNC7] its blood pressure of 130/80 down to 120/80 as normal, I think it would be safe to hypothesize that homocysteine ranges would be 5 to 9 or 10, and not have the absurd 5 to 15 range. *Reflect on this. The pharmaceutical manufacturer cannot patent the main nutrition supplements that deal with lowering homocysteine, and therein lies the problem.*

Don't wait until the scientific community takes their collective heads out of the sand and makes the general public aware of the serious risk factor of homocysteine.

It will be a win-win situation for you. If my hypothesis on homocysteine is right on causing my aortic and carotid artery stenosis, you can perhaps avoid them. If I am wrong, you'll still be healthier.

Source: The fabric of this chapter consists of abstracts and edited sources from:
Dr. Rodger Murphree
Dr. David W. Tanton, Ph.D.
Dr. Stephen Sinatra

Dr. Frederick Vagnini
Mark Hyman & Mark Liponis, M.D.'s
Life Extension Foundation.

Note: This chapter or any other chapter in this book is not meant to dispense medical advice or strategies for your health care. It is meant to raise your awareness to be pro-active to other health options which should be discussed with your health care professional.

CHAPTER 17

Elevated Glucose Spear

This chapter will not address type one diabetes, sometimes referred to as juvenile diabetes. This chapter is to address the possible onset of type two diabetes, sometimes referred to as adult onset diabetes. This happens in the majority of cases more often than not by ignoring the more subtle numbers of glucose readings just below or above 100 and repeated tests which creep above 100. This could conceivably indicate insulin resistance. *Insulin resistance [IR] is a condition in which the cells of the body become resistant to the effects of insulin, that is, the normal response to a given amount of insulin is reduced. As a result, higher levels of insulin are needed in order for insulin to have its effects. The resistance is seen with both the body's own insulin [endogenous] and if insulin is given through injections [exogenous].*

Insulin, therefore, has a profound effect on your glucose levels *which, if not kept within normal range, is a predecessor to diabetes*. The following are the ranges recommended by the American Diabetes Association:

Normal	- below 100 mg/dl
Pre-Diabetes	- 100 to 126 mg/dl
Diabetes	- above 126 mg/dl.

There are three different tests your doctor can use to determine whether you have pre-diabetes: the fasting plasma glucose test [FPG] or the oral glucose tolerance test [OGTT]. The blood glucose levels measured after these tests determine whether you have a normal metabolism, or whether you have pre-diabetes or diabetes. If your blood glucose level is abnormal following the FPG, you have impaired fasting glucose [IFG]; if your blood glucose level is abnormal following the OGTT, you have impaired glucose tolerance.

The 3rd test is Hemoglobin A1c. Measuring hemoglobin A1c is different from a single fasting blood glucose test from FFG or OGTT glucose test which is only a snapshot of one's current blood sugar level and is subject to daily variation. In contrast, the hemoglobin A1c test shows the bigger picture of a weighted average of blood sugar levels over the past three to four months.

<u>*Source*</u> for Hemoglobin A1c abstracted and edited from *Life Extension*, 4/08.

Diabetes is a silent stalker, and if you're over 45, overweight, and inactive, you're a prime target. It gives few overt warning signs. In fact, it is estimated that only half of those with this condition realize they have it, and its incidence is expected to double over the next ten years worldwide. In the United States alone over 16 million suffer with this condition, and 200,000 die every year of complications directly related to this disease.

<u>Diabetes is a fearsome disorder, yet one we take much too lightly. Few people flirting with border-line elevated blood sugar levels realize the urgency of controlling diabetes in its early stages.</u> *When your glucose levels are a little under or over 100 mg/dl, it's time to sit down with your health care professional for a way to lower it.* Most are unaware that diabetes is the

leading cause of blindness, kidney failure, and amputations in this country or that people who have diabetes are more likely to have-and die of-a heart attack or stroke than those with normal blood sugar metabolism. Nor do they recognize that diabetes is a primary contributor to erectile dysfunction [impotence] and dementia.

As a matter of fact, most people either don't know or tend to ignore the subtle warning signs of this devastating disease. It's time we all pull our heads out of the sand and look diabetes in the eye. Diabetes is in large part a disease of lifestyle. In 90 percent of all cases, it is both preventable and treatable-yet statistics clearly show that it is being neither prevented nor treated appropriately.

There are 20.8 million children and adults in the United States, or 7% of the population, who have diabetes. While an estimated 14.6 million have been diagnosed with diabetes, unfortunately, 6.2 million people [or nearly one-third] are unaware that they have the disease.

Type 2 diabetes is the most common form of diabetes. In type 2 diabetes, either the body does not produce enough insulin or the cells ignore the insulin. Insulin is necessary for the body to be able to use glucose for energy. When you eat food, the body breaks down all of the sugars, starches, proteins and carbohydrates [*all carbohydrates are not created equals as you will learn when you read the glycemic index*] turning them into glucose, which is the basic fuel for the cells in the body. Insulin takes the sugar from the blood into the cells. When glucose builds up in the blood instead of going into cells, your glucose levels rise. When they reach over 100 mg/LD, you are pre-diabetic.

Type 2 diabetes sneaks up on you. You don't suddenly lose weight or become excessively hungry and thirsty. It is usually discovered only during a routine blood test when a high fasting blood glucose reading, usually in the 150 to 300 mg/dl range is noted. *I feel if blood work were done several times a year you could be forewarned, that these numbers were creeping up and prevent yourself from becoming a diabetic victim. Track your blood work. That is how I noticed my readings were slowly creeping up over 100.*

The majority of the people in this group are:

- Overweight, with the distribution of weight most commonly in the abdominal area. Excess weight is a known factor in insulin resistance.
  Body Mass Index [BMI]: A BMI of 25 to 29.9 indicates a person is overweight. A person with a BMI of 30 or higher is considered obese.
  A way to determine your BMI is to multiply your weight in pounds by 704 and divide the result by height in inches squared. Example: 160 pounds x 704 = 112640 ÷ 5'7½" = 67.50 squared = 4556.25.
  112640 ÷ 4556.25 = 24.72 BMI.
- Inactive. Exercise enhances insulin sensitivity and reduces the risk of developing diabetes.
- Middle-aged. Once we hit our forties, our lifestyle indiscretions are no longer protected by the resilience of youth. Years of an unhealthy diet, extra pounds, and lack of exercise begin to take their toll and we succumb to degenerative

diseases-not only diabetes but also other diseases of aging such as heart disease, hypertension, and arthritis.

While diabetes and pre-diabetes occur in people of all ages and races, some groups have a higher risk for developing the disease than others. Diabetes is more common in African Americans, Latinos, Native Americans, and Asian Americans/Pacific Islanders, as well as the aged population. This means they are also at increased risk for developing pre-diabetes.

Syndrome X

In addition to being the driving force behind type 2 diabetes, insulin resistance is also part and parcel of a condition known as *syndrome X.* Identified in the mid-1980's by Stanford University researcher Gerald Reaven, MD, syndrome X is a cluster of disorders that includes obesity [particularly abdominal obesity], high blood pressure, elevated cholesterol and increased risk of heart disease and type 2 diabetes. Dr. Reaven, observing that these seemingly unrelated disorders cropped up so often in the same individuals, determined that the one underlying constant was glucose, both its level and its absorption.

Diabetes Chews Up the Body

Regardless of its cause-whether its inadequate production of insulin or an inability of cells to utilize it-excess glucose in the blood slowly but inexorably attacks cells throughout the body, binding to and altering proteins in a process called glycosylation that interferes with normal cellular function. Glucose is also converted into sorbitol, another form of sugar that accumulates in and damages cells. Excess blood sugar makes the blood thick and sticky, causing impaired circulation. Tissues that receive inadequate blood flow and become starved of oxygen and nutrients can sustain sometimes irreversible damage.

Another reason complications are so common in diabetes is because diabetes is nutritionally a wasting disease. As mentioned earlier, the diabetic condition causes dramatically increased urination as the kidneys attempt to get rid of excess glucose. Along with excess glucose, however, massive amounts of water-soluble vitamins and minerals also are lost. Yet incredibly, most white-coated experts specializing in diabetes make no attempt whatsoever to replace these nutrients, leaving their patients to suffer the inevitable consequences of massive nutritional deficiencies.

Numerous studies have shown that diabetics tend to have low cellular levels of magnesium, zinc, vitamins B6 and C, and other essential water-soluble nutrients. Is it any wonder that they are at increased risk for atherosclerosis, heart disease, and other degenerative conditions that have been definitively linked to nutritional deficiencies?

The combination of these processes puts diabetics at dramatically increased risk of premature death and disability. The areas of the body most profoundly affected by diabetes are the blood vessels, nerves, eyes, kidneys, and extremities. Diabetics are two to three times more likely to die from heart disease than those with normal blood sugar levels, and they are five times more likely to have a stroke. They are subject to vision problems such as glaucoma and cataracts, and diabetic retinopathy [*disease of the retina*], a leading cause of blindness. <u>Forty percent of all cases of kidney failure are attributed to this condition. Sixty to 70 percent of all diabetics have some form of nerve damage, and a majority of lower extremity amputations are performed.</u>

Prevention Is the Best Medicine

Although diabetes has probably been around for as long as our species has inhabited the earth [the condition is even present in some animals], the current epidemic is unprecedented in human history. There's a simple explanation for this phenomenon that can be summed up in three words: diet, inactivity, and obesity.

<u>Watch Your Diet</u>

One of the primary reasons we're seeing a worldwide glut of insulin-resistant diabetes is more and more emerging nations are adopting the Western diet that we've "enjoyed' for years. Indigenous diets of fresh fruits and vegetables, legumes, and whole grains are being replaced with processed, refined foods that have been stripped of their natural fiber and nutrients. Meat has become more prominent in the daily diet. And fast-food restaurants are springing up all over the globe.

In this country we've been eating a schizophrenic diet for years. In a futile effort to lose weight, we fill up on fat-free cookies and ice cream, which are nothing more than unhealthy refined carbohydrates. We've also become sugar junkies. According to U.S. Department of Agriculture statistics, Americans consume an average of 149 pounds of sweeteners a year-not counting the artificial sweeteners such as aspartame [NutraSweet and Equal] that we consume in over 7,000 products.

Excess fat is also a culprit, particularly saturated fats from meat and altered trans-fatty acids in processed foods. <u>As early as the 1920's it was demonstrated that a high-saturated-fat diet contributes to type 2 diabetes, as it not only causes weight gain-a risk factor in itself-but also decreases insulin sensitivity.</u>

<u>What you eat has a profound effect on your blood glucose levels and</u> your risk of developing insulin resistance and type 2 diabetes. <u>Refined carbohydrates and sugars are rapidly broken down into glucose, driving up blood sugar levels and placing an increased burden on normal metabolic processes.</u> On the other hand, vegetables, legumes, most fruits, and unrefined grains cause a slow, sustained release of glucose into the bloodstream. <u>Couple these slow burners with moderate amounts of low-fat protein and healthy monounsaturated and polyunsaturated fats, and you're on your way to balanced blood sugar control.</u>

Aim for moderate amounts of lean protein [20 percent of total calories], preferably from fish, poultry, tofu, egg whites, and legumes. Avoid saturated fats and trans fatty acids, found in margarine and other processed fats, and eat only healthy oils [20 percent of total calories], such as raw nuts and seeds, olive oil, and flaxseed oil. Make unprocessed carbohydrates [60 percent of total calories] the mainstay of your meals. Concentrate on fruits, vegetables, and legumes; avoid sugars and refined carbohydrates; and go easy on starchy carbohydrates such as bread, potatoes, and refined grains.

Exercise at Least Four Days a Week

Couple the current American diet, which packs a wallop of calories, with the sedentary lifestyle many have adopted, and what do you get? The fattening of America! One-third of Americans are obese, and obesity, particularly in the abdominal area, is a well-established risk factor for insulin resistance.

When you exercise, your muscles' energy requirements increase dramatically-they need ready access to glucose, which fuels the hungry muscle cells. Exercise appears to some degree to actually bypass the normal requirements for insulin. It increases the transport of glucose into the cells, not only while you are exercising but for hours afterwards. Thus it lowers blood glucose levels and also improves overall insulin sensitivity.

Researchers at Stanford and the University of California-Berkley who followed almost 6,000 men for 14 years determined that increased physical activity was effective in preventing type 2 diabetes. And it was especially protective for men with the highest risk of developing diabetes-those who were overweight or had a family history of diabetes.

Exercise also helps normalize weight, which is perhaps the single most important precipitating factor in reducing insulin resistance. To help avoid developing diabetes, I recommend at least 30 minutes of vigorous physical exercise four or more days per week. You don't have to run marathons-just get active. Brisk walking is one of the easiest activities for beginners, but the most important thing is to choose something you enjoy and stick with it.

Added Benefits to Exercise

"Researchers at Harvard University and Brigham Women's Hospital, writing in *Circulation: Journal of the American Heart Association*, report that weekly physical activity was associated with as much as 41% reduction in women's cardiovascular disease risk.

The researchers analyzed data on more than 27,000 female health care professionals, age 45 and older, who participated in the larger Women's Health Study on cardiovascular disease prevention. Participants all were apparently healthy and free of cardiovascular disease at the study's start. They provided blood samples and completed a questionnaire on physical activity, as well as follow-up questionnaires every six to 12 months over the course of more than 10 years.

The researchers found that as subjects exercised more, their risk for cardiovascular disease dropped accordingly: 27% for those whose activity measured 200-599 calories per week, 32% for these who burned 600-1,499 calories per week, and 41% for those who exercised the most, working off 1,500 calories or more per week."

Source: Tufts- Health & Nutrition Letter 1/08.

Take a High-Potency Multivitamin-Mineral Supplement Daily

Our current emphasis on refined, fatty foods is also responsible for nutritional deficiencies, as our consumption of vitamin-and mineral-rich fruits, vegetables, and whole grains has declined. It's ironic that in this land of plenty, millions suffer from inadequacies of certain important nutrients. Studies indicate that only a quarter of Americans get the recommended amount of magnesium, and intakes of zinc are also low. The average woman gets less than half the calcium she needs, and 58 percent of young women in the U.S. are iron deficient. Chief among the nutrients that are lost during the refining process is the trace mineral chromium, which enhances the action of insulin and also facilitates weight loss. It has been suggested that chromium deficiencies, which are common in this country, may play a role in the development of type 2 diabetes.

Dr. Whitaker recommends that everyone-even those who eat a good diet-take a high-potency multivitamin-mineral supplement every day. **Make sure your multivitamin contains "megadoses" of the nutrients that have been demonstrated to reduce risk of type 2 diabetes, namely vitamin C [1,700mg], vitamin E [800IU], vitamin B6 [75-100 mg],vitamin B12 [100-1,000 mcg], biotin [300 mcg], magnesium [500 mg], and chromium [200-400 mcg].** Think of your multivitamin supplement as insurance to counterbalance the inadequacies of your diet and compensate for the added nutrient requirements caused by our modern lifestyle. Believe me, it's the cheapest insurance policy you'll ever buy. *Speak to your health care professional for his recommendations for the multivitamins he recommends for you.*

Maintaining Normal Blood Sugar Levels Naturally

If you've been diagnosed with type 2 diabetes, the primary thrust of your medical management should be to get your blood glucose levels into the normal range. For most physicians, this means drug therapy. However, in over 25 years of treating thousands of type 2 diabetics at the Whitaker Wellness Institute, they have rarely found it necessary to prescribe drugs. For the majority of these patients, aggressive treatment with diet, exercise, weight loss, and natural agents that lower blood sugar is the ticket. In fact, by adopting this natural treatment program, a majority of the patients who come to the clinic already taking hypoglycemic drugs are successfully weaned from them.

Herbs That Lower Blood Glucose Levels

There are a number of herbs that have been studied for their ability to lower blood sugar. One is *Gymnema Sylvestre*, a plant native to India that, incredible as it may seem, appears to regenerate the insulin-producing beta cells in the pancreas. Gymnema has been demonstrated to lower blood sugar levels in both type 1 and type 2 diabetes. In a study of 22 type 2 diabetics, supplementation with this herb resulted in improved blood sugar control across the board, and

16 of the 22 patients were able to reduce their oral medications while five discontinued them altogether. The recommended dose of Gymnema is 400 mg per day.

Another herb utilized is banaba leaf [*Lagerstroemia speciosa L.*], which was only recently introduced in the US from Asia. Banaba leaf contains colosolic acid, which activates glucose transport into the cells, resulting in a reduction of blood sugar. In a 1998 Japanese placebo-controlled clinical trial, 24 diabetics were given a supplement containing banaba leaf or a placebo three times a day for four weeks. Significant blood sugar declines were observed in the individuals taking the herb [average 154.9 to 133.1 mg/dL]; there was little change in the placebo group. The suggested dose is 15 mg daily.

Other botanicals that improve control, albeit to a lesser degree, include bitter melon [*Momordica charantia*], Siberian ginseng, and those old kitchen favorites, basil, cinnamon, garlic, and onions. The most powerful natural glucose-lowering agents, however, are not plants but minerals.

Alpha-Lipoic Acid

Lipoic acid's best known biological effects are its use in diabetes. It has been used as a drug in the treatment of diabetes-related complications in Germany since 1960.

Several studies underscore the fact that dosages less than 600 mg per day are ineffective for diabetic neuropathy [*any and all disease or malfunction of the nerves*].

Chromium Facilitates the Action of Insulin

Chromium is a trace mineral that improves the action of insulin and helps move glucose and other nutrients into the cells. Its therapeutic value was first discovered in the 1950's, when researchers isolated a previously unknown substance from pork kidney. When they gave this substance to laboratory rats with glucose intolerance [a pre-diabetic form of insulin resistance], it caused such significant improvements that they named it *glucose tolerance factor [GTF]*. This unique compound was found to improve the activity of insulin and facilitate the uptake of glucose into the cells. Research intensified, and in 1959, the active ingredient in GTF was identified: Chromium. Chromium doesn't cause the body to make more insulin-it just helps make insulin work better.

At least 15 well-controlled clinical trials examining the effects of supplemental chromium on patients with diabetes, insulin resistance, and other blood sugar abnormalities have shown that this mineral improves glucose metabolism. In one recent study conducted by the US Department of Agriculture's Human Nutrition Research Center and Beijing Medical University, 180 type 2 diabetics were divided into three groups and given supplements containing 100 mcg chromium picolinate, 500 mcg chromium picolinate, or placebo, twice a day. No other changes were made in their medications, diets, or activity levels. When their blood glucose levels were tested after four months, the patients taking chromium had reductions in blood sugar, insulin, cholesterol, and glycated hemoglobin [a longer-term measure of blood sugar control]. Those taking 500 mcg per day generally had greater reductions than those taking the lower dose. Chromium has also been demonstrated to facilitate weight loss, which, as I explained earlier, is a powerful diabetic treatment in and of itself.

Vanadium Mimics Insulin

In Dr. W's opinion, the single most effective and intriguing weapon for addressing diabetes is vanadium. This unique trace mineral lowers blood sugar by mimicking insulin and improving the cells' sensitivity to insulin. Supplementation with vanadyl sulfate and other vanadium compounds markedly lowers fasting glucose and improves other measure of diabetes. In a number of animal studies this mineral has actually eliminated diabetes.

Human studies, although not as numerous, are also compelling. In a 1996 study, eight type 2 diabetics receiving 50 mg of vanadyl sulfate twice a day for four weeks, followed by a placebo for four weeks, were found to have a 20 percent reduction in average fasting blood sugar, which lasted well into the placebo period after the mineral was discontinued. The only reported adverse effect was minor gastrointestinal distress during the first few days of the study.

Vanadium is quite safe, even at doses of up to 400 mg per day. Don't be surprised if you hear rumors to the contrary. According to Dr. John McNeill, one of the world's leading experts on vanadium, these unfounded precautions are based on toxicity studies done by a single researcher and have never been replicated by anyone else. Dr. Whitaker and other physicians have utilized vanadyl sulfate with thousands of diabetic patients in doses of 100-150 mg per day with remarkable success and absolutely no adverse reactions, except for a slight GI distress in a few individuals.

Replace Lost Vitamins and Minerals

The key to the treatment of diabetes is twofold-control of blood glucose levels and, equally important, the prevention of complications. Yet while conventional physicians do attempt to stave off complications by keeping blood sugars in the normal range, they ignore the solid scientific research that supports the aggressive use of specific nutritional supplements for protections against the ravages of diabetes. One of the most obvious and inexcusable blind spots of conventional medicine and it can only be explained by an irrational bias against nutritional supplementation.

As Dr. Whitaker explained earlier, diabetes is a nutritionally wasting disease. Massive amounts of nutrients are lost as the kidneys rid the body of excess glucose by increasing urination, so the first step is replacement of these lost nutrients. Among the most significant losses are the B-complex vitamins, and many diabetics have suboptimal cellular levels of these vital nutrients. Vitamins B6, B12, and biotin improve insulin sensitivity and also help prevent diabetic complications, particularly neuropathy, which is present in almost half of all diabetics. Supplementation is imperative, with recommended doses of 75 mg vitamin B6, 100-1,000 mcg of B12, 300 mcg of biotin, and an array of other B-complex vitamins.

Diabetics also tend to have low levels of magnesium, and those with the lowest levels are most likely to have diabetic retinopathy [*disease of the retina*] and other eye problems. Dr.

Whitaker suggests supplementing with a minimum of 500 mg of magnesium per day, balanced with 1,000 mg of calcium.

Antioxidants are also important. Vitamin C, the most active antioxidant in our water-based tissues, lowers levels of sorbitol, the sugar that collects in and damages cells of the eyes, kidneys or nerves. Vitamin E, the body's premier fat-soluble antioxidant, improves glucose control and protects blood vessels and nerves from free-radical damage, which is accelerated by the diabetic condition. Studies have shown that high doses of supplemental vitamin E may even reverse damage to nerves caused by diabetes and protect against diabetic cataracts and atherosclerosis. Supplementation with both of these antioxidants is associated with a reduced risk of diabetic retinopathy. Dr. Whitaker recommends diabetics take 2,500 mg of vitamin C and 800 IU of vitamin E daily.

Nutritional deficiencies are the easiest aspect of diabetic management as they simply require supplementing with copious amounts of nutrients to compensate for the drain caused by the diabetic condition. The simplest way to do this is to take a daily multivitamin and mineral supplement. Although the bulk of the vitamins and minerals discussed in this report are included in most multivitamin and mineral supplements, the amount of each nutrient they contain is often woefully inadequate. Most one-a-day brands contain only the government's recommended daily allowances [RDAs], which, in Dr. Whitaker's opinion and based on available scientific literature, are absurdly low. Read labels carefully and look for a high-potency formula, or augment individual nutrients to achieve the therapeutic doses recommended in this report.

Source abstracted and edited from Dr. Julian Whitakers, Special Welcome report "Reverse Diabetes Damage and Normalize Blood Sugar Naturally". Dr. Whitaker Julian is the director of The Whitaker Wellness Institution, Newport Beach, CA.

THE GLYCEMIC INDEX

The best way to keep insulin and blood sugar levels low is to eat carbohydrates that rank low on the glycemic index. This index shows the rate at which carbohydrates break down as sugar or glucose in the bloodstream. Foods with a high-glycemic index release glucose into the bloodstream quickly, causing a rapid rise in blood sugar and a subsequent rise in insulin. Low-glycemic foods usually contain more fiber and release glucose into the bloodstream at a slower rate.

When you eat high-glycemic foods, enjoy them – just be sure to mix them with healthy fats, protein and lower-glycemic carbs so you can prevent insulin spikes. If you do that. You'll not only preserve your insulin, but your HDL "good" cholesterol will become higher and you'll protect your blood vessels.

Some significant information for using a glycemic index when planning on what you eat:
- low GI means a smaller rise in blood sugar and can help control established diabetes
- low GI diets can help people lose weight and lower blood lipids (fats)
- low GI diets can improve the body's sensitivity to insulin

- high GI stimulate insulin surges which can cause people to eat 60-70% more calories at the following meal
- high GI elevate insulin and blood glucose
- high GI stimulate fat storage

In researching glycemic index foods the majority were ranked using number reference which, I felt, was not consumer friendly.

I have listed them in a more consumer friendly ranking:
- desirable foods, <u>low GI</u>, 39 percent and below
- moderately desirable, <u>moderate GI</u>, 40 percent to 69 percent
- less desirable foods, high GI, 70 percent and up

Note: There's a 10-15% variation of these rankings depending on the standards used to define the foods.

Desirable Foods, low GI, 39% or below

Breads:
Coarse European-style, whole grain wheat of rye pita bread, cracked or sprouted whole wheat.

Cereals:
Compact noodle-like high bran cereals (All-Bran, Fiber One), coarse oatmeal, porridge, coarse whole grain (Kashi), cereal mixed with Psyllium (Fiberwise)

Pasta, Grains and Starchy Vegetables:
pasta (all types
barley, bulgur,
buckwheat (kasha)
couscous, kidney beans dry,
lentils, black-eyed peas,
chick peas, kidney beans,
lima beans, peas, sweet potato,
yam (soybeans lowest)
Most vegetables, including: artichokes, asparagus, broccoli, carrots, cauliflower, celery, cucumbers, egg plant, green beans, lettuce, peas, peppers, spinach, tomatoes

Milk Products & Dairy:
Skim, 1%, cottage cheese (lowfat or regular), buttermilk, low-fat plain yogurt, low-fat fruited yogurt, low-fat frozen yogurt (artificial sweetener),
Egg substitutes (cholesterol free) cottage cheese

Fruit:
Most fruit and natural fruit juices, including apple, berries, cantaloupe, cherries, grapefruit, honeydew, oranges, pears, grapes, peaches, applesauce (cherries, plums and grapefruit lowest)

Meats:
Shellfish, "white" fish (cod, flounder, trout, tuna in water), chicken, turkey, cornish hen, venison (white meat, no skin)

Soups:
Lentil
Tomato

Moderately Desirable Foods, moderate GI, 40% to 60%

Breads:
100% stone ground whole wheat,
Pumpernickel,
100% whole grain, rye crisp, cracker

Cereals:
Grape-nut cereal, medium-fine grain oatmeal
(5-minute variety), All-Bran, Kellogg's All-
Bran fruit and oats

Pasta, Grains and Starchy Vegetables:
Rice, boiled, potato, corn, navy beans, kidney
beans (canned), baked beans, beets, bulgur,
pasta

Milk Products & Dairy:
2% milk, cheese, regular plain yogurt

Fruit:
Banana, kiwi, mango, papaya, orange, pears,
grapes, apples, grapefruit, plum, apricot,
peach, grapes

Meats:
Higher fat fish (salmon, herring), lean cuts of
beef, pork, veal, low-fat imitation luncheon
meat, low-fat cheese, eggs

Less Desirable Foods, high GI, 70% and up

Breads:
White bread, most commercial whole wheat
breads, English muffins, bagel, French
bread, most commercial matzoh, Melba
toast, Cheerios, pumpernickel, donuts

Cereals:
Corn flakes, puffed rice, puffed wheat, flaked
cereals, instant "Quick" or precooked
cereals. Oatbran, rolled oats. Shredded
wheat, Muesli, cream of wheat, millet,
cornmeal, Special K, , buckwheat, grape-
nuts, Rice Crispies

Pasta, Grains and Starchy Vegetables:
Instant rice, brown rice, instant pre-cooked
grains, baked potato, microwaved potato,
instant potato, Winter squash (acorn,
butternut), parsnips, French fries, waffles,
buckwheat, stone wheat, couscous, sweet
corn, beets, parsnips

Milk Products & Dairy:
Whole milk, ice milk, ice cream, yogurt
sweetened with sugar, low-fat frozen
desserts with sugar added, low-fat and
regular frozen yogurt with sugar added.
Tofu ice cream.

Fruit:
Pineapple, banana, dates, fruit juices
sweetened with sugar, raisins, watermelon.

Meats:
Most cuts of beef, pork, lamb, hot dogs
(including "low-fat" versions), cheese,
luncheon meats.

Miscellaneous:
All bakery goods, all candy, chips, honey , ice
cream, peanut butter, pop corn, pretzels,
split pea soup

Source: abstracted and edited, Dr. Ann de Wees Allen
Glycemic Research Institute

Steer Clear of Artificial Sweeteners. Aspartame [NutraSweet], neotame, acesulfame
potassium, saccharin, sucralose, and dihydrochalcones are artificial sweeteners consumed by
two-thirds of the adult population and are a significant component of our diets. They are in

many packaged foods, artificially sweetened foods, gum, candy, sodas, drinks, and mints. Read the labels and look for those names. *Sugars have been linked to some forms of cancer.*

A number of studies have shown that aspartame ingestion may actually lead to increased food and calorie intake. This is likely because artificial sweeteners make your body produce insulin by making it think sugar is on the way. As a consequence, your body tells you to eat more sugar to balance your insulin level. Artificial sweeteners do nothing to help in this regard. They do not act as sugar does and do not balance your insulin. As a result, you end up with excess insulin in your body, so you end up eating more food to take care of this problem. This whole pattern disrupts your appetite control system in serious ways. What's worse, it can lead to insulin resistance, which has many serious health consequences. *Studies have linked Aspartame to possible Multiple Sclerosis and dementia.*

Insulin resistance leads to high glucose readings. That is why you should consult with your health care professional when your glucose levels are approaching 100 or slightly over to create a strategy to reverse the trend.

Abbreviated Elevated Glucose Summary Recommendations

1. Keep glucose well under 100 mg/dl.
2. Quit smoking.
3. Exercise.
4. Overweight, BMI.
5. Take high potency multi-vitamins/mineral supplements daily.
6. Herbs that lower blood glucose levels:
   a. Gymnema Sylvestre.
   b. Banaba leaf.
7. Supplements that are helpful.
   a. Chromium picolinate.
   b. Alpha-lipoic acid.
   c. Biotin.
8. Vanadium mimics insulin.
9. Follow recommendations of glycemic index.
10. Stay away from artificial sweeteners.

Avandia Warning

If you have high levels of glucose and your doctor wants to prescribe Avandia [rosiglitazone], my research revealed:

• Steven E. Nissen, M.D. [a very noted doctor with the Cleveland Clinic – see Bio below], the lead investigator of a meta-analysis – as reported in the *New England Journal of Medicine 2007*, 356:2457-2471] a 43% relative excess hazard of myocardial infarction – *heart attack [MI]*- found with Avandia compared with controls in his analyses of 42 randomized trials.

• There is a running controversy between Dr. Nissen and the manufacturer of Avandia – Glaxo SmithKline – that Dr. Nissen is [figuratively speaking] cherry picking. *If you will recall, in Chapter Four on trials and studies – a meta analysis is from many trials – this was from 42 trials.* Thus, Glaxo SmithKline's Philip Home, professor of diabetes medicine, University of Newcastle upon Tyne, U.K., funded by Glaxo SmithKline he is "data snooping on quite a big scale." Released interim data on a study called Record [Rosiglitazone Evaluated for Cardiac Outcome and Regulation of glycemia in diabetes] which basically disagrees with Dr. Nissen's meta-analysis. [Dr. Nissen is the chairman of the Cleveland Clinic Hospitals' Department of Cardiovascular Medicine. *U.S. News & World Report* consistently names Cleveland Clinic as one of the Nation's best hospitals. They have 1,500 full-time salaried physicians on staff. They had approximately 54,000 hospital admissions to Cleveland Clinic in 2005.]

I don't know about you, but his warnings get my complete attention.

Lowering blood pressure may raise glucose anatomy of HcTZ [Hydrochlorothiazide, a diuretic.] Some studies have shown that there is indeed a higher risk of elevated glucose, others have not confirmed this finding.

Dr. Asqual Getaneh, an assistant clinical professor of Medicine at Columbia University, New York City, where she specializes in diabetes and obesity, states: "Thiazide diuretics have proven beneficial to people with high blood pressure and are among the best, safest, and least expensive of blood pressure drugs. The use of beta-blockers [which are also prescribed to treat high blood pressure] along with thiazide diuretics can, however, increase blood glucose levels. It is possible that hydrochlorothiazide increases the production of glucose from the liver, and because beta-blockers limit the absorption of glucose into cells, the use of these medicines in tandem can raise glucose levels significantly enough to cause diabetes." *Author: It can also raise your serum creatinine.*

Note: This chapter or any other chapter in this book is not meant to dispense medical advice or strategies for your health care. It is meant to raise your awareness to be pro-active to other health options which should be discussed with your health care professional.

CHAPTER 18

Blood Viscosity Spear

Thin Blood Keeps Your Heart Healthy
[from an abstract by Dr. Stephen Sinatra in *Heart, Health & Nutrition*, 2/06]

"Blood is thicker than water" is an old saw expressing the importance of family ties. But in the medical world, you don't want thick blood.

In June 2004, I first reported to you about blood viscosity – meaning thickness – and how the flow and the protective mechanisms interact inside arterial tissue. Blood viscosity, an overlooked element in blood tests, has become an emerging major marker for identifying your risk for atherosclerosis.

The thicker your blood, the slower it flows through your circulatory system to bring vital nutrients to the cells of your body, and the greater the risk of forming clots. You want your blood to be thin like wine, not sludgy like ketchup.

Many times in cardiology, we actually extract blood from high-risk patients in order to thin their blood and prevent a heart attack. And, of course, Coumadin has been widely used as a standard medication to thin the blood and help prevent clotting.

Knowing the critical nature of this, you can only imagine my excitement to have recently learned about a newly developed device that measures blood thickness. The Rheolog, as it's called, takes a small amount of a patient's blood, and within three minutes returns an analysis in the form of a thrombogenic potential number. The higher the number, the thicker your blood."

- **The Importance of a Blood Viscosity Measurement**

"Knowing your blood viscosity [*the resistance of a fluid flowing* freely] provides you with a critical tool in determining the efficiency and health of your cardiovascular system and the onset or acceleration of your cardiovascular condition.

Even if you have already been diagnosed, knowledge of your blood viscosity will allow you to make significant treatment decisions toward improving your quality of life and outcome.

The role that blood viscosity plays in cardiovascular health is substantial. Since the cardiovascular system is a closed system, the viscosity or thickness of what the heart is pumping is of critical importance. Blood is a complex, shear-thinning fluid which can be five times thicker when the heart is at diastole than at systole – as much as ten times thicker in patients with severely pathological blood flow. Blood viscosity affects not only how hard the heart has to work to circulate the blood, but also affects the level of stress, injury and inflammation the blood causes to the arteries. The thicker the blood is, the more the abrasion and damage it does to the arteries resulting in arterial damage, hardening of the arteries, growth of atherosclerosis or plaque rupture.

Understanding the viscosity of your blood allows you to know well in advance the long-term prognosis for your cardiovascular health and the ability to design and begin a treatment regimen with your doctor before further damage is done.

Source: Rheologics, Inc., Uuchlan Ave., Suite 414, Exton, PA, 19341.

- "The Rheolog® Scanning Capillary Viscometer is an investigational device that requires a minimally invasive sampling procedure presenting no significant risk: the blood sample is not returned to the patient's body, nor does the Rheolog by design or intention introduce energy into a subject. The Rheolog is not used as a diagnostic procedure without confirmation of the diagnosis by another medically established product or procedure. The Rheolog device is considered to be exempt from the requirements of the IDE regulation, in accordance with the provisionals specified in 21 CFR §12.2 and 812.5.

Whole blood viscosity measurements can be performed ex vivo [*in the living body*] at the point-of-care or in vitro [*in a test tube*] in a laboratory setting. In the latter case, two [2] blood samples of 3 mL are collected using standard lavender-top [EDTA] vacutainer vials, stored between 2 and 7 deg C, and measured within a period of 4 days or less after specimen collection. Inquiries may be directed to The Blood Clinic at 866-300-5958 to participate in a blood viscosity testing." For more information visit their website www.thebloodclinic.com.

Kenneth R. Kensey, M.D. with Carol A. Turkington, authors of *The Blood Thinner Cure* book.

An Abstract about thick blood from their book:

"Most doctors will tell you that arthrosclerosis is caused by a chemical process: cholesterol and other chemicals in the blood clog the arteries. Yet, even patients with extremely high cholesterol have athosclerosis in only a few of their arteries. If athosclerosis were caused *only* by things such as a high-fat diet or high cholesterol, then we would expect to see *all* of the arteries in your body affected – because all of the arteries are exposed to the same blood, but that doesn't happen.

I believe atherosclerosis occurs because your heart has pumped thickened blood at too high a pressure for too long, which *physically* injures certain regions of the arterial system, making the arteries hard and inflexible. Within these hardened regions, blood flow becomes turbulent, and the blood then begins to erode your arteries at specific sites. These sites are often where your arteries branch."

- **Why Arteries Harden**

"For a long time, many scientists thought that hardened arteries and plaques didn't have anything to do with each other – that they occurred independently and that they were perhaps two entirely different processes. Dr. Kenneth R. Kensey does not agree.

Dr. Kensey believes that arteries harden first, and this in turn triggers the formation of blockages – they are directly related. Dr. Kensey feels that all the risk factors for atherosclerosis have one common denominator: your heart is working too hard because of thickened, sticky blood – what he calls "the sludge factor."

When blood is pumped through the flexible arteries of your body, the arteries bulge with each pulsing heartbeat as a way of accommodating the pressure. A child's arteries are very soft and expand effortlessly as the heart pumps, making it easy for the blood to move throughout the body smoothly and quietly. As you age, blood pressure begins to rise, and your blood gets thicker. The blood vessel must cope with higher and higher pressure and thicker and thicker blood. In certain regions this overstretches and injures your arteries. As your blood pressure continues to rise and your blood gets thicker, the heart must work harder to pump the blood. This in turn forces the arteries in the same regions to overstretch even more. This overstretching injures the arteries, which respond to this injury by getting harder to avoid further overstretching.

In recent years, many studies have suggested – and Dr. Kensey agrees – that atherosclerosis begins with an *injury* to their artery lining that leads to the clogging. What Dr. Kensey suggests is that the hardening of the artery wall [arteriosclerosis] is caused by a *physical* [*mechanical*] injury, not a chemical one. While Dr, Kensey believes that diet, lifestyle, and heredity all play a role in mechanically injuring the arteries, the primary cause of artery hardening, as well as the clogging itself, is the way your arteries adapt to this mechanical injury."
Source: Dr. Kenneth R. Kensey.

My personal experience in trying to deal with the possibility that my blood might be too thick:

As I mentioned in chapter one, because I relied on my internist and good friend of over 20 years as my medical *Holy Grail – if you have a better reason than mine for being your own health advocate, I'd like to hear it.* – I have aortic value and right internal carotid artery stenosis.

I am sure many of you, as I, have read about people having heart attacks and/or strokes due to blood clots. I always wondered to myself, why don't they have a test [*which they didn't*] for blood viscosity to prevent this type of an event.

After my diagnosis I felt I might be in that profile for clotting and I asked my new former cardiologist – "remember," I said, "I saw five different cardiologists" [in 6/05] "to put me on Plavix "– [*I remembered reading Dr. Sinatra's first article [6/04] on thick blood which causes blood to clot, and by using Plavix I would prevent a heart attack or stroke*].

My wife and I and some friends were playing golf [*approximately 8 months later*] in Naples, Florida. The hotel we were staying at delivered *U.S.A. Today* at our hotel door every A.M.

An article in *USA Today* on 3/13/06 [their source: American College of Cardiology, printed online in *The New England Journal of Medicine*] stated that a recent study raised a safety concern. It showed that Plavix plus aspirin [*I was not taking aspirin, I was using Ginkgo Biloba, another natural blood thinner*] nearly doubled the heart disease death rate among patients who had not yet had a heart attack or stroke and were using it prophylactically [*as I was*], but who had multiple risk factors such as high blood pressure and diabetes – *Oh, did I forget to mention I had high blood pressure but it is now under control with medications 116/65].*

They went on to mention it proved safe and effective in patients who had strokes and heart attacks but not on patients using it prophylactically as I was.

On my return from the golf trip, I made an appointment with my present and still cardiologist, Dr. Vagnini, in Garden City, New York.

I showed him the *USA Today* article regarding the Plavix study. He told me the AMA has not released any changes on the use of Plavix. I told him, 'Fred, forget about the AMA. Suppose you were taking it, what would you do?" He said, "I would discontinue its use."

By a fortunate coincidence of fate Dr. Vagnini had just been sent a machine by Rheologics to use in a study to measure blood viscosity.

I took the test on 3/17/06 the same day [*while I was still on Plavix*]. I got the results in less than 5 minutes on a computer read-out on a comparison graph. The median number they recommended was 23. I was at just under 11 [*the lower the number, the better*].

7/20/06 – I was off Plavix approximately 13 days. [*I called the drug manufacturer; they said your body would clear it in ten days.*]
Their median number still being 23, I was at 18.

7/24/06 – I increased the omega-3, I was taking before the first test on 3/17/06, from 1½ grams to 3½ grams.
Their median number still being at 23, I was now at 13.5.

I was now off of Plavix and 9.05 points better than the recommended median of 23.

I also recently had two dental implants done and had no bleeding problems and only discontinued taking omega-3, one week prior to the procedure.

I highly recommend you discuss this test with your doctor and arrange to take it ASAP.

Note: This chapter or any other chapter in this book is not meant to dispense medical advice or strategies for your health care. It is meant to raise your awareness to be pro-active to other health options which should be discussed with your health care professional.

CHAPTER 19

Hypertension Spear

Even people without hypertension may need to watch their blood pressure.

"If Americans don't start taking their blood pressure seriously, we're likely to end up with a country where the vast majority have to worry about high blood pressure," says Ramachandran Vasan, M.D., a researcher for the Framingham Heart Study, the nation's longest-running study of cardiac risk factors.

High blood pressure wreaks havoc with the heart and the arteries, greatly increasing the risk of heart attack, stroke, and heart and kidney failure. Hypertension also increases the risk of Alzheimer's disease and possibly subtle mental declines. And it may thin the bones, since the elevated pressure apparently increases calcium excretion.

Today more than one out of four American adults have high blood pressure. Dr. Vasan considers that an epidemic, and notes that it's getting worse. Another 15 to 25 percent of the population have "high-normal" blood pressure, just below the official cutoff for hypertension. Recent Framingham results show that this group faces a much higher cardiovascular risk than previously thought – high enough to warrant aggressive lifestyle changes. Moreover, the danger of cardiovascular disease rises steadily with blood-pressure levels; thus many people in the "normal" range face a greater risk than those with lower, "optimal" levels [see box, below]. Indeed, some who currently have normal blood pressure could be headed for serious trouble, thanks to inactive lifestyles and other unhealthy habits.

Why normal blood pressure may not be best.			10-YEAR CARDIOVASCULAR RISK [PERCENT]	
BLOOD PRESSURE CATEGORY	SYSTOLIC [MM HG]	DIASTOLIC [MM HG]	MEN	WOMEN
Optimal	Less than 120	Less than 80	5.8	1.9
Normal but not optimal	120 to 129	80 to 84	7.6	2.8
High-normal	130 to 139	85 to 89	10.1	4.4
High	140 or more	90 or more	about 12.1	about 5.3

Beware of blood pressure spikes especially in and out of the recommended range.

An announcement made on CBS in the segment they call TIMELINE, where brief health announcements are sometimes made, claims that blood pressure could vary up to 40% depending upon the time of day and season, is a prescription for a possible stroke or heart attack, especially if you have other cardio risk factors. This is a very critical reason to work on getting your blood pressure in the recommended blood pressure category.

Note: source was abstracted and edited.

Why Heart Patients Should Aim for Lower Pressures

If you have heart disease, simply avoiding hypertension probably isn't enough, a recent Cleveland Clinic study suggests.

To stunt the growth of plaque inside your coronary arteries and avoid a heart attack, bypass surgery, angioplasty or other major event, reach for new depths, suggests Steven E. Nissen, M.D., chair of the Department of Cardiovascular Medicine at Cleveland Clinic and president of the American College of Cardiology.

Hypertension means systolic [high number] pressures of 140 millimeters of mercury or higher and diastolic [low number] pressures of 90 or higher. But evidence is mounting that these numbers are particularly risky for heart patients. "If your home-monitored systolic blood pressures are marginal – say between 130 and 140 – that's probably too high," Dr. Nissen says.

He led a study, published in 2004, called CAMELOT, exploring whether blood pressure medications could reduce heart patients' risks. "The most provocative finding was than when we lowered systolic pressures by about five millimeters of mercury, we saw a relative reduction of more than 30 percent in cardiovascular events," he says [November 10, 2004, *Journal of the American Medical Association*]. For the new study, the CAMELOT researchers used an ultrasound probe to measure changes in the volume of plaque in the walls of heart vessels over a two-year period.

"We found that getting your systolic pressure below 120 is necessary for maximum benefit in slowing plaque growth," Dr. Nissen says [August 15, 2006, *Journal of the American College of Cardiology*].

Source: *Harvard Heart Letter.*

But for many people the problem is reversible. In the past two years, a string of important studies have shown that several commonly recommended lifestyle measures – healthy diet, regular exercise, and weight loss – can dramatically reduce blood pressure, especially when combined. Those steps create the biggest reductions in people who have high blood pressure, but they may also have significant benefits in those with high-normal or even normal but not optimal levels.

Why normal isn't optimal

Officially, hypertension isn't diagnosed until systolic blood pressure [the upper number] reaches 140 millimeters of mercury [mm Hg] or diastolic pressure [the lower number] reaches 90 mm Hg. But there's no magic point at which blood pressure becomes dangerous. Rather, the risk of heart attack and stroke increases steadily as blood pressure rises.

A recent 25-year study of nearly 13,000 men from seven countries found that heart-attack risk increases by about 30 percent for every 10 mm Hg rise in systolic pressure and every 5 mm Hg rises in diastolic pressure, even within the normal range. Other studies have found similar increases in women and have suggested that stroke risk also rises steadily with blood pressure.

By the time those levels reach high-normal – 130 to 139 mm Hg systolic or 85 to 89 mm Hg diastolic – the risk is considerable, especially for older people.

Dr. David G. Williams, M.D. states in his *Alternatives* newsletter [summer 2004, vol. 9, no. 29], "as we age, <u>our blood vessels lose some of their elasticity</u>, which often leads to higher systolic [top number] blood pressure.

In Dr. Stephen Sinatra's *Heart, Health & Nutrition* 1/2006, in an abstract of a conversation with Charles C. Mary III, M.D., director of the Mary Clinic in New Orleans:

"A Conversation with Charles Mary III, M.D.

Sinatra: Do you find that high-dosage vitamin C is beneficial for cardiovascular patients in your practice?

Mary: Absolutely. The cardiology profession overlooks this fundamental vitamin. You can't have venous or arterial health without it. <u>You cannot make enough good collagen to keep blood vessel tissue flexible, vital, and strong</u>."

The conclusion I draw from these two isolated statements: Vitamin C is an extremely important nutrient to be taking.

Among Framingham participants over age 65 who had high-normal pressure [130-139-85-89], the 10-year risk of heart attack or stroke was 25 percent for men and 18 percent for women – roughly double the rate of people with optimal blood pressure. According to guidelines adopted in 1999 by the World Health Organization and several European countries, that's substantial enough to warrant antihypertensive drugs. Our medical consultants won't go that far, since studies have not yet proven the benefit of drug therapy for this group. But they agree that aggressive lifestyle changes are definitely warranted.

Younger people with high-normal [130-139-85-89] blood pressure face a lower 10-year risk – 4 percent for women and 8 percent for men – but need to be just as concerned. By age 65, they'll likely face even higher risk than those who develop high-normal pressure later in life.

Lifestyle changes may also be justified for people whose blood pressure is normal but not optimal. <u>Individuals with a systolic pressure of 120 to 129 mm Hg or a diastolic of 80 to 84 have 30 to 50 percent higher cardiovascular risk than people with lower, optimal readings of less than 120/80 mm Hg</u>. More important, "it's safer and easier to keep blood pressure down in the first place than to try reducing it later," says Frank Sacks, M.D., at the Harvard School of Public Health. Such efforts are especially important in black people [who are more likely than whites to die of hypertension-related complications] as well as in those with other cardiac risk factors, such as high cholesterol levels, excess weight [especially around the waist], and diabetes or prediabetic blood-sugar levels.

Unfortunately, other recent findings from <u>Framingham show that the vast majority of us are headed in the wrong direction. More than half of people ages 55 to 65 and nearly two-thirds</u>

of those over age 65 are likely to develop hypertension within the next 10 years. And the dangers posed by high blood pressure don't diminish with advancing age, as doctors once thought.

"If you want to buck that trend, you need to act now," says Dr. Sacks.

Eat the Right Foods

Population studies have long shown that people who eat lots of produce and little fat have lower blood pressure than other people. But studies of the individual elements thought to possibly provide that benefit – including calcium, fiber, magnesium, potassium, various antioxidant vitamins and nutrients, and a low fat intake – have found either no or only small benefits from boosting the intake of specific nutrients.

A few years ago, researchers at five leading hospitals around the country took a different tack, by testing the whole diet rather than its individual components. The results of the trial known as DASH [Dietary Approaches to Stop Hypertension], demonstrated that a diet high in fruits, vegetables, whole grains, and low-fat dairy products could indeed substantially lower blood pressure levels. "It may be that the particular nutrients work better when they're all together, or that there's something else in whole foods that also helps," says Dr. Sacks.

Last year, Sacks and his colleagues published the results of a follow-up trial confirming the original results. Overall, the two studies show that people with hypertension who adopt the diet can expect to lower their blood pressure an average of about 8 mm Hg systolic and 4 mm Hg diastolic – an amount rivaling that achieved by some anti-hypertensive drugs. Those without hypertension can expect declines of about 4 mm Hg systolic and 2.5 mm Hg diastolic. Those numbers may not sound like a lot, but anything that causes and presumably maintains even small blood pressure declines is important, since it counters most people's tendency toward rising levels.

Some experts have worried that the DASH results couldn't be repeated outside of the study, since the trial participants had all their meals carefully prepared for them according to strict guidelines. But in May, British researchers showed that a similar diet can indeed work in the real world. Nutritionists merely explained the principles of the diet to some 345 volunteers and provided simple recipes to get them started. After six months, the volunteers achieved blood-pressure 130-139-85-89.

Just a DASH of Salt

In addition to confirming the original finding, the second DASH trial investigated whether cutting back on salt can lower blood pressure further. While government guidelines have long urged all Americans to consume less sodium, the scientific consensus behind that recommendation isn't very strong, especially for those individuals who don't have hypertension. The new DASH study has helped clarify the effects of sodium.

Volunteers were assigned to either a regular diet or the DASH diet. Every month, the sodium content of both diets was changed, so they consumed either 3,500 milligrams [mg] a day, the U.S. average; 2,400 mg a day, the government-recommended ceiling; or 1,500 mg a day, an extremely low amount. On average, blood pressure fell in sync with sodium reduction in both diets, and in all subgroups, including people with or without hypertension, blacks or whites, young or old, and normal weight or obesity.

The benefits were especially striking when combined with the DASH diet, and in people who had hypertension or an increased risk of developing it. For example, people with high blood pressure on the DASH diet who consumed the least sodium dropped their systolic reading an additional 4.9 mm Hg compared with those who consumed the most, for a total decline of 11.5 mm Hg. In black people, the low-sodium diet boosted the effect of the DASH diet by 3.6 mm Hg, for a total decline of 9.6 mm Hg.

However, getting to the low sodium levels used in the study poses practical difficulties. Taste is the least of them, since in most people the craving for salt disappears after a few weeks. But only about 15 percent of dietary sodium comes from the salt shaker. About 10 percent is a natural part of food and 75 percent is added to food during processing or cooking. Prepared canned or frozen foods as well as restaurant fare tend to be especially salt-laden. So getting down to the 1,500 mg [my level] would require people to cook nearly all their food at home, from scratch.

Simply adopting the DASH diet will likely reduce sodium intake close to the 2,400 mg level. Some of the experts we spoke with said that everyone should make the extra effort needed to cut back to 1,500 mg per day; others felt that almost no one needs to go that far. We think the evidence justifies a compromise position: The effort is definitely worthwhile for individuals who have hypertension, probably justified for black people and those with high-normal blood pressure or a family history of hypertension, and possibly helpful for some people with normal but not optimal blood pressure. Since some people respond dramatically to sodium, you don't necessarily have to reach the 1,500 mg goal to see a meaningful decline, although the less sodium you consume, the lower your blood pressure will likely go. Conversely, not everyone responds to a low-sodium diet. So you may not need to continue the extra effort if you don't see an improvement after several months of serious effort.

Added Measures

As the DASH-plus-low-sodium diet shows, people who make multiple lifestyle changes can achieve substantial blood-pressure reductions. Those who add the changes described below can expect even larger declines – which are comparable to those seen in the DASH trial.

While the DASH diet requires substantial dietary changes for most people, notably eating significantly more produce and less meat, the British trial showed that people can do it on their own. The effort is certainly worthwhile. The diet not only reduces blood pressure but also helps lower cholesterol levels and has numerous other health benefits, including a possible reduction in cancer risk. For more on the diet, see the box below.

The new blood pressure diet

The DASH diet can seem daunting, because it includes 7 to 12 daily servings of fruits and vegetables, depending on how large and active you are. [It also includes 6 to 13 servings of grains, preferably whole; 2 to 4 servings of low-fat dairy products; 1 to 3 servings of meat, poultry or fish; 2 to 4 servings of oil or other fats; and 3 to 7 servings a week of nuts, seeds or beans.] If you want to cut back on salt, the diet can be even more imposing. However, serving sizes are quite small, as the following examples show. And a number of steps can help you lower your salt intake.

Serving sizes:
- *Vegetables:* ½ cup of cooked or raw chopped vegetables; 1 cup of raw leafy vegetables; or 6 ounces of juice.
- *Fruit:* 1 medium apple, pear, orange, or banana; ½ cup of fresh, frozen, or canned fruit; ¼ cup of dried fruit; or 6 ounces of juice.
- *Grains:* 1 slice of bread; ½ cup of cold, dry cereal, cooked rice, or pasta.
- *Dairy:* 1 cup of nonfat or low-fat milk or 1½ ounces of low-fat or part-skim cheese.
- *Meat, poultry, or fish:* a 3-ounce chunk, roughly the size of a deck of cards.
- *Nuts, seeds, and beans:* ½ cup [1½ ounces] of nuts; 2 tablespoons of seeds; or ½ cup of cooked beans.

Salt tips
To cut back on salt:
- Flavor foods with lemon, lime, wine, vinegar, or a variety of herbs and spices instead of salt.
- Eat more whole, unprocessed foods; choose fewer processed, canned and convenience foods.
- Limit cured foods [such as bacon and ham], foods packed in brine [such as pickles, olives, and sauerkraut], and condiments [such as mustard, horseradish, ketchup, and Worcestershire, soy, or teriyaki sauces].
- Look for products labeled "sodium free" [5 milligrams or less of sodium per serving]; "very low sodium" [35% milligrams or less]; or 'low sodium" [140 milligrams or less].

Salt Sampler

The Institute of Medicine has unveiled new guidelines for salt intake.

Current recommendation: **2,400 mg**
New Recommendation: **1,500 mg**
What average person eats: **4,000 mg**

Sodium Content of Some Foods
• Dill pickle [large]: **1,900 mg**
• Top Ramen Creamy Chicken [1package]: **1,300 mg**
• McDonald's Big Mac: **1,050 mg**
• McDonald's French Fries [medium]: **290 mg**
• Campbell's Select Chicken Vegetable soup [1/2 can]: **830 mg**
• Prego Mini Meatball pasta sauce [1/2 cup]: **660 mg**
• Hot dog [plain]: **540 mg**
• Chocolate cake [packaged, 4-inch slice]: **360 mg**
• Bran muffin/corn flakes: **300 mg**
• Peanuts, salted [1/4 cup]: **272 mg**
• Soda: **25-50 mg**

Source: University of Minnesota Extension Service;
Campbell Soup Company; McDonald's.

This diet would sharply reduce cardiovascular risk. Researchers estimate that every 2-point decline in systolic pressure lowers coronary risk by 5 percent and stroke risk by 8 percent.

• **Work out.** A recent analysis of 54 exercise trials concluded that moderately paced aerobic workouts, such as brisk walking, can lower blood pressure in people with hypertension by an average of 5 mm Hg systolic and 4 mm Hg diastolic. Black people had even larger declines.'

Such workouts reduce blood pressure at least as effectively as vigorous exercise does. People with hypertension should avoid strenuous workouts, at least until they get clearance from their doctor. Strength training may also help – but people with hypertension should avoid holding their breath or straining, which can cause potentially dangerous spikes in blood pressure.

• **Lose weight.** Both the DASH and the exercise studies probably underestimate the potential benefits of diet and exercise for many people. That's because the exercise regimens generally burned too few calories to cause weight loss, and the DASH diet provided just enough calories to prevent it. Presumably, consuming fewer calories or exercising more would lead to weight loss. And that clearly reduces blood pressure.

Obesity also raises blood pressure, blood cholesterol levels, triglyceride levels, lowers HDL ["good"] cholesterol levels, and increases insulin resistance. Insulin is a hormone responsible for delivering glucose [blood sugar] into the cells where it is used as fuel. Excess fat cells can block insulin receptors and increase the risk of sugar deposited in the artery instead of the intended cells. This can set up a chain reaction that results in arteriosclerosis and heart disease. Increased fat cells also cause the heart and cardiovascular system to work harder. <u>It is estimated that it takes one mile of capillaries [smallest blood vessels] to supply each pound of fat. What if you are 10 to 20 pounds overweight? This translates to 10 to 20 extra miles of capillaries that must be serviced by the heart.</u>

However, losing just 10 pounds of weight results in an average decreased systolic pressure of seven points and a drop of five points in diastolic pressure. A one point drop in diastolic pressure results in a three percent decreased risk of heart disease and a seven percent decreased risk of stroke.

A weight gain of 10% can increase systolic blood pressure by 6.5 points. Total cholesterol typically increases 12 points for every 10% increase in weight gain.

• **Go easy on NSAIDs.** Regular use of no steroidal anti-inflammatory drugs [NSAIDs], such as ibuprofen [Advil, Motrin], naproxen [Aleve], and ketoprofen [Orudis-KT], appears to boost blood pressure slightly, especially in older people and those with hypertension. The drugs may also blunt the action of certain antihypertensive medications, particularly beta-blockers. So use NSAIDs regularly only when the benefits clearly outweigh that and other risks, such as stomach bleeding – in most people with severe arthritis, for example. [Regular use of low-dose aspirin does not appear to pose the same risk.]

• **Drink moderately, if at all.** Heavy drinking raises blood pressure. But moderate imbibing – no more than one drink a day for women, two for men – does not raise pressure and may even lower it slightly by relaxing the blood vessels, according to one study. But don't start drinking for that reason.

• **Relax.** <u>You may want to try stress reducing techniques, such as yoga, meditation, or cognitive-behavioral therapy, especially if you're high strung or under a lot of stress.</u> While the evidence that such steps lower blood pressure is mixed, studies that focused on hypertensive or very stressed individuals generally have shown a benefit.

• **Don't smoke.** Stopping smoking lowers blood pressure only slightly. But it cuts heart-attack risk substantially.

• **Control snoring.** People with sleep apnea – almost invariably heavy snorers – repeatedly stop breathing for up to a minute while they sleep. That causes blood pressure to spike,. Researchers at the Mayo Clinic in Rochester, Minn., recently showed that those brief but repeated nocturnal elevations can eventually damage the arteries and perhaps contribute to chronic hypertension. A recent study in the *Journal of the American Medical Association of more than 6,000 adults did indeed link severe snoring with a 45-percent increase in the likelihood of developing hypertension.*

To control snoring, try losing weight, sleeping on your side, and avoiding alcohol and sleeping pills. If it persists, consider seeing a sleep specialist, who can diagnose sleep apnea and, if necessary, suggest other treatments.

Summing up

Lifestyle changes can help people with hypertension eliminate or reduce their need for medication. People with either high-normal or normal but not optimal blood-pressure risk may benefit, too.

The table below describes the four most effective steps for lowering blood pressure. Other potentially helpful measures include reducing stress, cutting back on nonsteroidal anti-inflammatory drugs, avoiding excessive alcohol consumption, and stopping smoking. The more steps you take, the greater the likely reductions will be.

<u>Source</u>: *Consumer Reports on Health* 9/02

WHAT WORKS		
Advice	**Details**	**Drop in Systolic Blood Pressure**
Lose excess weight	For every 20 pounds you lose	5 to 26 points
Follow a DASH diet	Eat a lower fat diet rich in vegetables, fruits, low dairy foods	8 to 14 points
Exercise daily	Get 30 minutes a day of aerobic activity [like brisk walking]	4 to 9 points
Limit Sodium	Eat no more than 2400 mg a day [1500 mg is better]	2 to 8 points
Limit alcohol	Have no more than 2 drinks a day [men] 1 drink a day [women]. [1 drink = 12 oz. beer, 5 oz. wine, or 1.5 oz. 80-proof whiskey]	2 to 4 points

Source: The Seventh Report of the Joint National Committee on Prevention, Detection, Evaluation, and Treatment of High Blood Pressure.

Your Adrenal Gland and Hypertension

Although we often talk about high blood pressure as if it were a disease, it really isn't. It is a symptom of trouble somewhere in the body. High blood pressure usually accompanies excess weight, declining kidney function, and arteriosclerosis, the narrowing and stiffening of blood vessels. One often overlooked cause of high blood pressure is a malfunction of the adrenal gland.

The adrenals [once called the supraenal] are triangular glands that perch atop each kidney. They churn out hormones that affect the stress response and the immune system. They also make aldosterone. This hormone helps manage the body's balance of water, sodium, and potassium. Too much aldosterone makes the kidneys hang on to sodium and water and flush potassium into the urine. The extra fluid ends up in the bloodstream. This forces the heart to push harder to propel blood on its journey through thousands of miles of blood vessels, which raises blood pressure. Overproduction of aldosterone is known as aldosteronism.

Overactive adrenal glands were once thought to be a relatively rare cause of high blood pressure. That view is changing. A number of studies, including a large Italian study published last fall in the *Journal of the American College of Cardiology*, suggests that overproduction of aldosterone accounts for up to 5 in 100 cases of newly diagnosed high blood pressure. In people with resistant hypertension, aldosterone contributes to 20 cases in 100. And there is growing evidence that excess aldosterone adds to heart disease in other ways as well.

Beyond blood pressure

Too much aldosterone may do more than boost blood pressure. Experiments in animals show that excess aldosterone triggers inflammation in blood vessels; turns down production of nitric oxide, a molecule needed to relax blood vessel walls; and dulls the activity of blood pressure "thermostats" known as baroreceptors. These receptors keep blood pressure steady by instantly changing the heart's output or the tension on blood vessels.

Studies in humans have shown that using the drug spironolactone [generic Aldactone] to block aldosterone's activity improves survival in people with advanced heart failure. Eplerenone [Inspra] does the same thing for heart attack survivors with damage to the left ventricle, the heart's main pumping chamber. Work under way is exploring whether aldosterone-blocking medications should play a larger role in controlling heart disease.

Source: Harvard Health Letter 4/07.

Low Vitamin D levels linked with Increased Blood Pressure

Another new study points to a link between vitamin D levels and cardiovascular health, and may help explain why hypertension seems to afflict more black Americans than other ethnic groups.

Using data from the Third US National Health and Nutrition Examination Survey, researchers found that individuals with the lowest vitamin D levels had slightly higher blood pressure. Non-Hispanic white Americans had the highest vitamin D blood levels, followed by Mexican Americans, while non-Hispanic black Americans had the lowest levels.

"This finding may have public health significance, as vitamin D levels can easily, and cheaply, be increased by a modest increase in sun exposure or vitamin D supplementation," researchers noted in the *American Journal of Hypertension*.

Many public health experts now advise that all adults should increase their vitamin D intake to at least 1,000 IU per day and should regularly monitor their blood levels.

Source: Scragg, R., Sowers, M., Bell C. Serum 25-hydroxyvitamin D; ethnicity, and blood pressure in the Third National Health and Nutrition Examination Survey, *American Hypertens.* 2007, July 20(7):713-9.

- In the book *Wilson's Syndrome* (1991/1996), Dr. E. Denis Wilson explains Hypothyroid condition is one possible influence on blood pressure – *this issue could be addressed with a simple blood test.*
- In the book *Drug-Free Approach to Health Care*, the author, David W. Tanton, Ph.D. states what conditions in the blood cause high blood pressure.
  - Restriction in the kidneys
  - Buildup of arterial plaque causing loss of elasticity in the blood vessels
  - Blood viscosity [which was discussed in Chapter 18].

Dr. Tanton's book goes on to state (abstracted form): The depletion [or a deficiency] of the following nutrients can result in high blood pressure:

- Vitamin B-1
- Vitamin B-2
- Vitamin B-6
- Choline
- Vitamin E
- Calcium
- Magnesium
- Potassium
- Essential fatty acids (EFAs)
- Co Q 10
- Sugar is another contributing factor to high blood pressure and the creation of plaque.

Lowering blood pressure may raise glucose anatomy of HcTZ [Hydrochlorothiazide, a diuretic.] Some studies have shown that there is indeed a higher risk of elevated glucose, others have not confirmed this finding.

Dr. Asqual Getaneh, an assistant clinical professor of Medicine at Columbia University, New York City, where she specializes in diabetes and obesity, states: "Thiazide diuretics have proven beneficial to people with high blood pressure and are among the best, safest, and least expensive of blood pressure drugs. The use of beta-blockers [which are also prescribed to treat high blood pressure] along with thiazide diuretics can, however, increase blood glucose levels. It is possible that hydrochlorothiazide increases the production of glucose from the liver, and because beta-blockers limit the absorption of glucose into cells, the use of these medicines in tandem can raise glucose levels significantly enough to cause diabetes." *Author: It can also raise your serum creatinine.*

Note: This chapter or any other chapter in this book is not meant to dispense medical advice or strategies for your health care. It is meant to raise your awareness to be pro-active to other health options which should be discussed with your health care professional.

CHAPTER 20

I Use Baselines, and I am not Talking about Baseball;
Giving this Blood May Save Your Life.

For over 4,000 years, the leech has been a familiar remedy with Greek and Roman physicians using the application of this clever blood sucking invertebrate [*lacking backbone*].

In modern medicine, leeches have proven useful in microsurgery in which surgeons work for hours to reconnect an appendage. Doctors have found that an operation can fail because tiny blood vessels become clogged. They have found that using leeches is the most efficient way to remove the clogged blood from the tiny vessels. Eating healthy, exercising, and supplements with the appropriate nutrients are only part of the strategy needed to reach optimal health and well-being.

Annual blood screening can help give you a complete picture [*which I believe should be more frequent if you have health issues, and not by using leeches*] and is one of the most important step aging adults can take. With blood tests, you can be forewarned of many critical changes in your body before they manifest themselves in your body. That is one of the basic purposes for which your doctor orders them. Sadly, most annual medical check-ups involve the physician ordering only routine blood tests. In my opinion, *they should be the cornerstone of any preventive steps you can take in your health* care, there are no routine blood tests – *as you read on and will see by Bio Reference Labs list.* Each doctor has his preference of the type of tests he orders. Let's hope you have the right doctor.

The doctor I go to has his preference of the blood screenings he wants, but since we are partners in my health care, I discuss additional tests I would like.

Folks, when time is of the essence and a serious threat to your life meets you head-on, and lifestyle changes won't give you a quick response, you must turn to prescription drugs because of their quick response to the problem your body requires. On the other hand, if you consider the preventative approach as I do, you should discuss these additional tests with your doctor and in the event there are indications you have a problem, you may be able to turn to nutritional supplements and let the healing powers of Mother Nature do what they were meant to do. If they require the additional boost of prescription drugs, your doctor will use them in conjunction with the supplements.

I also believe in baselining on my Excel program by establishing your blood chemistry levels prior to starting on a strategy by taking supplements and/or prescription drugs prescribed by your doctor. As an example:

- Raise your HDL
- Lower your LDL
- Lower your triglycerides
- Lower your glucose.

By using this method, I can track my general health in these areas and be forewarned as well of any positive or negative effects [*indicated by the lab ranges*] of any medications and nutritional supplements I am taking.

Before I recommend the additional blood screenings you should ask your doctor to add to his preference list for you, I would briefly like to discuss test results and doctors' diagnoses.

Don't let the expression before you go through that procedure, "get a second medical opinion," be limited to a doctor's diagnosis. You should also include labs he uses upon which he bases his diagnosis on and seek another doctor who uses a different lab for a second opinion.

Let me give you a few examples:

Newsday, 10/3/07.
"A lab error by CBL Path Medical Lab, Rye Brook, NY was responsible for a double mastectomy."

Newsday, 2005.
"Lab error by Quest Labs [one of the largest labs in the country] led to a lumpectomy and 25 radiation treatments."

My personal experience with Quest Labs pales by experience.

During my consultation with Dr. Sinatra he advised me to strive for a Co Q 10 level of a minimum of 2.5 as that was a therapeutic range for someone with my conditions.

1st. Quest Lab report came back for my Co Q 10 value stating, "Unfrozen specimen received. Test requires a frozen specimen," by Metametric Medical Research in Norcross, GA, the lab Quest had sent my specimen to for Co Q 10 evaluation.

2nd Quest lab report came in with a Co Q 10 range of 1.6. [*I never went back to give a second specimen for that bogus report.*]

3rd Lab report *I chose another lab]* I got from Enzo Labs. It was 0.4.

I relied on the Enzo Lab report of 0.4 instead of the bogus report from Quest.

I adjusted my dosage accordingly and my Co Q 10 range was 3.4 in a subsequent test from my new lab. [*See Chapter 9 and 20 to see the importance of Co Q 10 to your heart.*]

By receiving a copy of all my tests I was able to catch this lab error early and make the necessary corrections to avoid any problems.

To add insult to injury, they billed me for it. It took me over 3 months of phone calls and letters to get Quest to admit their error and send me a credit for the charge.

Therefore, I feel it is in your health's own best interest to get a copy of all your reports to catch any irregularities so they can be nipped in the bud.

As far as the two unfortunate women I mentioned earlier, had they had a copy of their first lab's reports and challenged them, perhaps their doctor would have obtained different labs' opinions and the tragedies could have been avoided.

My recommendations for blood screening are not in order of medical priority.

In looking over the printed form by Bio Reference Laboratories for blood work my doctor fills out, I did a double-take. Here is the variety of blood screenings they offer:

Chemistry profiles	8*
Microbiology	11*
Alphabetical Listings, individual tests	69*
Other special tests	9*

*Each of these includes several or more components.

You can readily see that one size fits all does not apply. That's why all doctors have their preferences as to the tests they order for you.

The following recommended tests that I add on to my doctor's preference list are based on my own personal experience tracking my blood work and my research. I recommend them for people who have known CAD [or Coronary Artery Disease] or have risk factors for CAD such as smoking, diabetes, cholesterol and hypertension. [Note: some of these tests may appear on your doctor's preference list.]

BNP. One Study in the *Journal of American Medical Association* found that a higher level of an amino acid chain, called NT-proBNP, in blood plasma was associated with a higher incidence of heart failure and death from a cardiac event. It is considered a better predictor of mortality in people at moderate to high risk for a cardiovascular event.

Calcium. There is more calcium in the body than any other mineral. It works together with phosphorus [present in every cell in the body] for healthy bones and teeth. Calcium and magnesium work together for cardiovascular health. When taking calcium supplements, always take with it Vitamin D. Calcium is needed for adequate control of muscular contractions, transmission of nerve impulses and blood clotting. High levels could increase the risk of urinary tract infections.

Researches found in the nurses' study of 85,764 women after adjusting for cardiovascular disease, that women with the lowest levels of calcium had a greater risk for stroke.

An over-retention can cause hypercalcemia [elevated levels of calcium in the blood], which can result in fatigue, depression, confusion, anorexia, nausea, vomiting, constipation, pancreatitis or increased urination. If it is chronic, it can result in renal [kidney] stones or bladder stones and abnormal heart rhythms. Severe hypercalcemia is considered a medical emergency and cardiac arrest can result.

Source: Earl Mendells' Vitamin Bible, Life Extension, and Wikipedia.

Coenzyme Q10 Serum [CoQ10] – is a fat-soluble cofactor essential for energy-producing metabolic pathways and for the proper functioning of the mitochondrial oxidative system. With insufficient CoQ10, the electron transfer activity of the mitochondria decreases, resulting in a net failure to produce the energy necessary to run the cell. Tissues with high energy demand have even greater demands for CoQ10. For example, heart muscle, which continually exerts a pumping action for an entire lifetime, has an immense need for this cofactor. Studies demonstrate the effectiveness of supplemental coenzyme Q10 in cardiomyopathy, myocardial dysfunction and congestive heart failure. CoQ10 is also a powerful antioxidant like vitamin E and C, and thus serves the role of neutralizing excess free radicals. It is now well established that the control of excessive free radical activity is the key in preventing/delaying the progression of degenerative diseases.

Therapeutic information: Serum CoQ10 measurements such as this test mirror bioavailable levels. If Serum CoQ10 is low, it can be increased by supplementing according to the following: 38 to 100 mg daily for prevention of cardiovascular or periodontal disease and for patients taking HMNG-CoA reductase inhibitors, 98 to 100 mg daily for angina pectoris, cardiac arrhythmia, hypertension and moderate gingival disease, 100 to 360 mg daily for congestive heart failure and dilated cardiomyopathy. CoQ10 is best absorbed when taken with a balanced meal.

Source: Sinatra, S. Coenzyme Q10 and the Heart.

Fibrinogen is a coagulation-type protein that determines the stickiness of your blood by enabling your platelets to stick together. You need adequate fibrinogen levels to stop bleeding when you are cut, but higher than normal fibrinogen levels have been associated with too much blood clotting – and you know what overly clumpy blood can do.

A high fibrinogen level over 300 mg/dl is considered undesirable and is considered an independent risk for heart disease and by itself can cause the abrupt formation of a coronary thrombosis.

You can lower your risk for high fibrinogen levels:

- Stop smoking. It can shoot your levels through the roof.
- Dr. Sinatra's natural blood thinners are: ginger, omega-3 fish oil, gingko biloba, Vitamin E and bromelain.
  Source: The Sinatra Health Report 2/01.

Glucose. This test is critically important in detecting early stage metabolic syndrome, diabetes and coronary artery disease and could be another red flag for you to start to address issues like weight loss and diet, and a conference with your health care professional. See Chapter 17, "Elevated Glucose Spear," for the three types of tests available.

Homocysteine – is an inflammatory biomarker that raises your risk factor for a heart attack or stroke. Even if you take folic acid you may still have dangerously high levels of this artery-clotting metabolic debris. In most cases it can be lowered with the correct amounts of folic acid, V-6, B-12 and TMG. *Source: Life Extension.*

Hs-CRP – highly sensitive C-Reactive Protein.
In the year 2000, *The New England Journal of Medicine* published a study reporting that C-reactive protein levels [hs-CRP], which is another inflammatory bio-marker, can help predict future heart risks even in people with "low risk" cardiac profiles. In fact, the study showed that hs-CRP was twice as effective as a standard cholesterol test in predicting heart attacks and strokes.
Source: *Toxic Blood Syndrome.*

Investigators at the Brigham & Women's Hospital in Boston monitored 28,263 apparently healthy post-menopausal women over a three-year period. In addition to looking at CRP, the researchers evaluated homocysteine and a variety of cholesterol and lipid measurements. Of the 12 markers measured, hs-CRP was the strongest predictor of future cardiac events.

There is a common thread in the majority of modifications one can do to correct these issues: stop smoking [*if you do*], exercise [*if you don't*], eat correctly [*for some that would be another book*], take targeted nutritional supplements such as CoQ10, omega-3 fish oil, and consult your health professional.

Potassium. Potassium works with sodium to regulate the body's water balance and normalize heart rhythms.

Nerve and muscle functions suffer when the sodium-potassium balance is off and it is thus important in maintaining fluid and electrolyte [sodium, potassium, calcium, magnesium, chloride, phosphate and hydrogen carbonate] balance in the body.

As you can see, potassium is quite important to be in the proper lab range with your potassium levels because potassium levels affect your heart rhythms.

On one of my visits to "Dr. Feel Good," my former cardiologist reviewing my latest labs, he said in his warmest Gestapo voice, "Paul, if your potassium levels go any higher, you'll drop dead of a heart attack. See my nurse on the way out, she will give you a list of foods with a high potassium level so you can avoid them."

When I got home to peruse the list [*let me say this before I go any further – when it's from the doctor, that's the gold standard: "not so!"*], the omissions on his list of "foods to avoid," compared to the book, *Healthy Diet Calorie Counter* by Kirsten Hartvig, were glaring.

His intimidating warning, coupled with his cavalier perception of "foods to avoid" certainly lowered his medical credibility with me.

Since potassium is a mineral and is present in all fruits, nuts and seeds, vegetables, meats, fish, dairy products, fats and oils, grains, cereal, breads, soups, sauces and drinks, and you have a predisposition to have high potassium levels, it would be in your best interest to find a doctor who has a nutritionist on his staff to properly advise you regarding this issue.

PSA-Prostate-specific Antigen. A PSA level over 2.5 NG/ML, or a PSA doubling time [the time required for PSA value to double] of less than 12 years may be cause for concern.

The American Cancer Society recommends annual PSA testing for men beginning at age 50, even in the absence of prostate abnormalities and also include a digital rectal exam.

Men in high-risk groups should begin screening at age 45 [high risk groups include African-American men, and men whose brothers, fathers, or sons had been diagnosed with prostate cancer under age 60].

Lipid Peroxides.
What are Lipid Peroxides? In its efforts to produce the chemical energy to power your cells and fight infection, your body makes harmful chemicals called free radicals. Breakdown of your body cell membranes by free radicals leads to the formation of lipid peroxides. Antioxidants protect you against this process, and the lipid peroxide test tells you if you have enough of these antioxidants in your system. High levels of lipid peroxides are associated with cancer, heart disease, stroke and aging.

What does my Lipid Peroxide Result Mean? If your lipid peroxides are high, your body is failing to control the rate of formation of free radicals. You can increase your protection by taking vitamin E and C, selenium, beta-carotene, and bioflavonoids. Many products are available that offer combinations of these and other antioxidants that may be beneficial.

These test results are not for the diagnosis of diseases. They are intended to provide nutritional guidelines to qualified healthcare professionals with full knowledge of patient history and concerns to assist in their design of an appropriate healthcare program. [*Source: Metametric Clinical Laboratory*]

Lipid Profile. The chemistry panel provides information of the status of your cardiovascular system:
- Total cholesterol
- HDL [high density lipoprotein]
- LDL [low-density lipoprotein]
- Triglycerides, cholesterol/HDL ratio, LDL, CHOL calculated,
- or the new VAP [expanded cholesterol test].

VAP [expanded cholesterol test]. There is a revolutionary new cholesterol test. It is able to identify whether cholesterol problems are in the genes or only due to improper diet and lack of exercise. In 90% of abnormal cholesterol problem, proper diet, exercise, and supplementation can correct the imbalance even when it is genetic. Standard cholesterol tests usually include total cholesterol, HDL, LDL, and triglycerides scores. The VAP test includes all of these traditional measures and a detailed breakdown of the start forms of HDL and LDL particles present in your blood. New research is showing that some HDL and LDL particles are big and fluffy [these particles are better] and some particles are small and dense [these particles are much more dangerous]. The test quantifies all of these measures for you. It also indicates which pattern you are. Your pattern refers to your genetic risk factor for heart disease. You will either be a pattern A [best], B [worst], or AB [in the middle].

Lipoprotein [a] – Lp[a].
Lp[a] is a cholesterol particle that causes inflammation and clogging of blood vessels because of its repair properties, and is actually an LDL particle that has an adhesive protein surrounding it, giving it sticky properties.

Under normal circumstances, Lp[a] is one of the most effective repair molecules in your artery walls. In the presence of Vitamin C deficiency, however, Lp[a] can become one of the most dangerous risk factors for atherosclerosis.

In a study published in *Circulation* [a journal published by the American Heart Association], researchers gathered data from 27 different studies which collectively tracked more than 5,200 people who had either survived a heart attack or been diagnosed with heart disease. The average age of the study participants was 50.

The study clearly shows that there is a direct connection between LP[a] elevation and an increased risk of heart disease.

Dr. Sinatra suggests the nutritional supplements you can take to lower it are Vitamin C, CoQ10, L Carnitine, omega-3 fish oil and Niacin B-3.

You should seek the advice of your health professional for the proper dosages.
Source: Dr. Sinatra, *Heart Sense 12/02.*

Testosterone [Free]. Testosterone is a steroid hormone derived from cholesterol. In men, levels normally decline with age, dropping to approximately 65% of young adult levels by age 75. Following menopause, the levels of testosterone also decrease.

Adult Testosterone Effects. Adult testosterone [estrogen] effects are more clearly demonstrable in males than in females, but are likely important to both sexes. Some of these effects may decline as testosterone levels decline in the latter decades of adult life.
- Maintenance of muscle mass and strength
- Maintenance of bone density and strength
- Libido and clitoral engorgement/penile erection frequency
- Mental and physical energy
- The most recent and reliable studies have shown that testosterone does not cause prostate cancer, but that it can increase the rate of speed of any existing prostate cancer. Recent studies have also shown its importance in maintaining cardiovascular health.
- A lack of testosterone can lead to statistically significant increase in the likelihood of cardiovascular disease [CVD], and type 2 diabetes [one-third of all men with type 2 diabetes

have low testosterone]. Low testosterone can cause osteoporosis in males. A lack of testosterone has been shown to be associated with increased adipose fat, obesity and a difficulty in losing excess weight and has been strongly associated with depression. Most alarming is the recent evidence/studies that have shown that a lack of testosterone greatly increases mortality rates in men over 50.

If your tests reveal low testosterone levels, you should be screened for hemochromatosis [excessive iron] and have insulin levels, blood sugar, fibrinogen and LP[a] checked. These risk factors for heart disease may be – and often are – elevated when testosterone is low.

There are many strategies you can discuss with your doctor to help to correct this issue [e.g., keep your weight down, don't smoke, cut out or cut down on alcohol]. Vitamin C, E and zinc cruciferous vegetables like broccoli and Brussels sprouts are helpful. Avoid over-the-counter drugs like Tylenol, which can interfere with the liver's function. If you must take drugs like "statins," antibiotics, beta blockers or Coumadin, stop eating grapefruit. It not only affects the efficacy of the medications, it turns on the aromatase enzyme complex in the brain, fat and testes. When there's an overload of this enzyme, testosterone levels literally fall through the floor.

Source: Wikipedia, Stephen Sinatra, M.D.

How much vitamin D do you need?

Vitamin D – Abstracts from *Scientific American*

Key Concepts
- Vitamin D, long associated only with its role in bone formation, is actually active throughout the human body, powerfully influencing immune system responses and cell defenses.
- It can be obtained from food or manufactured by human skin exposed to sunlight. Measures of vitamin D levels show, however, that many people have too little of it circulating in their blood to protect health.
- Clear associations between low vitamin D levels and cancers, autoimmunity, infectious diseases and other conditions suggest that current daily intake recommendations for this critical nutrient needs revision.

Sources of Vitamin D

Vitamins D_3 and D_2 occur naturally in some foods, and both versions of the vitamin are added to certain "fortified" products. Foods provide relatively small doses of D compared with amounts made by the skin in response to UVB light. [IU = international units.]

- Cod-liver oil [1 tbsp.]: 1,360 IU D_3.
- Cooked tuna, sardines, mackerel or salmon [3-3.5 oz.]: 200-360 UI D_3.
- Shiitake mushrooms [fresh, 3.5 oz.: 100 UI D_2 [dried, 3.5 oz.]: 1,600 IU D_2.
- Egg yolk: 20 IU D_3 or D_2.

- Fortified dairy products, orange juice or cereals [one serving]: 60-100 IU D_3 or D_2.
- Full body exposure to UVB [12 to 15 minutes at midday in summer, fair skin]: 10,000 IU D_3.

Tissues Affected by Vitamin D

The VDR receptor protein is found in many body tissues as well as circulating immune cells, indicating a role for active vitamin D in those lactations. The list below includes some of the tissues and cells where 1.25D action has been established:

- Bone
- Brain
- Breast
- Fat
- Intestine
- Immune cells
- Kidneys
- Liver
- Nerves
- Pancreas
- Parathyroid gland
- Prostate
- Skin keratinocytes

D Makes a Difference

Growing evidence suggests that chronically low levels of vitamin D raises a person's risk for certain major illnesses. Examples of findings based on a population's blood serum D levels or UV exposure include;

- 30% to 50% higher risk for breast, prostate and colon cancers at serum 25D levels below 20 ng/ml.
- Five times higher risk of ovarian cancer among women living at high latitudes [for example Norway and Iceland] than women living in equatorial regions.
- 77% lower risk for all cancers among Nebraska women age 55 and older taking 1,100 IU of D_3 daily over a three-year period compared with a placebo group.
- 62% lower risk for multiple sclerosis at serum 25D levels above 40 ng/ml than at 25 ng/ml or less.
- 80% lower lifetime risk for autoimmune [type 1] diabetes in Finnish children given 2,000 IU of D_3 daily during first year of life.

How Much 25D is Desirable?

Estimates of vitamin D available to the body are based on measurements of 25D concentrations in blood serum. Levels between 30 and 45 nanograms per milliliter of serum are considered minimally sufficient for bone health, although some beneficial cellular responses to D are optimized at higher concentrations. Below 30 ng/ml, health risks increase; above 150 ng/ml, excess calcium build-up in blood and tissues and symptoms of toxicity are possible.

B-12 [*CoBalamin*] – Source: Abstract from *Earl Mendell's Vitamin Bible*

<u>What It Can Do for You</u>:

Form and regenerate red blood cells, thereby preventing anemia.
- Promote growth and increase appetite in children.
- Increase energy.
- Maintain a healthy nervous system.
- Properly utilize fats, carbohydrates, and protein.
- Relieve irritability.
- Improve concentration, memory, and balance.

<u>Facts</u>
- Water soluble and effective in very small doses.
- Commonly known as the "red vitamin," also cyanocobalamin.
- Cyanocolabamin is the commercially available form of vitamin B12 used in vitamin pills.
- Measured in micrograms [mcg.]
- The only vitamin that contains essential mineral elements.
- Not well assimilated through the stomach [should be taken sublingual – under tongue]. Needs to be combined with calcium during absorption to properly benefit body.
- Recommended adult dose is 50 mcg., to 100 mcg. Suggested for pregnant women and 2.6 mcg. For nursing mothers.
- A diet low in B1 and high in folic acids [such as a vegetarian diet] often hides a vitamin-B12 deficiency.
- A properly functioning thyroid gland helps B12 absorption. Symptoms of B12 deficiency may take more than five years to appear after body stores have been depleted.
- In the human diet, vitamin B12 is supplied primarily by animal products, since plant foods [with minor exceptions] don't contain it.

Source: Abstract from Dr. Sinatra's *Heart Sense*, 12/99

<u>A recent British study showed that patients with Alzheimer's had lower levels of folate and B12. I can't stress enough the importance of B vitamins.</u> They're critical for brain health because they support nerve function. The problem is, many elderly people [65 and above] typically don't absorb B12 because of age-related changes in the digestive tract caused by increased growth of intestinal bacteria that impairs their ability to absorb Vitamin B-12 from food. They should take a sublingual form of vitamin B12.

Source: Abstract from the authors of *Ultra Prevention*, Mark Hyman and Mark Liponis, M.D.

Vegetarians who do not take supplements cannot get enough vitamin B12, since plants do not produce it [and vitamin B12 is essential for memory, nerve function, energy metabolism, regulation of homocysteine, red blood cell formation, and much more].

B12 – Earl Mendell recommends Supplements:

"Because B12 is not absorbed well through the stomach, I recommend the sublingual form of the vitamin, or the time-release form – accompanied by sorbitol – so that it can be assimilated in the small intestine.

Supplements are available in a variety of strengths from 50 mcg. To 2,000 mcg.

Doctors routinely give vitamin B-12 injections. If there is a severe indication of deficiency or extreme fatigue, this method might be the supplementation that's called for.

Daily dosages most often used are 5 to 100 mcg."

Note: This chapter or any other chapter in this book is not meant to dispense medical advice or strategies for your health care. It is meant to raise your awareness to be pro-active to other health options which should be discussed with your health care professional.

CHAPTER 21

You don't have to do Crunches to Keep your Intestinal Tract in Shape [although, it wouldn't hurt]. You Need Pro-Biotics.

Doctors are over-prescribing antibiotics [which are only effective against bacteria, not viruses], and destroy intestinal flora.

CHICAGO [AP] – Doctors wrote 12 million antibiotic prescriptions in a single year for colds, bronchitis and other respiratory infections against which the drugs are almost always useless, a study found.

- Such indiscriminate use of antibiotics has contributed to the emergence of drug-resistant bacteria, a growing problem in the United States, the researchers said.

- More that 90 percent of upper respiratory infections, including bronchitis and colds, are caused by a virus [*and not bacteria*] and are therefore impervious to antibiotics, researchers noted in Wednesday's *Journal of the American Medical Association.*

- Doctors usually know this, but studies have suggested they may yield to pressure from patients – or what they perceive to be the patient's expectations – to prescribe a drug, even if it is unlikely to help.

- "Every time we use an antibiotic, we run the risk of promoting antibiotic resistance, or drug resistance, by bacteria," said the lead author, Dr. Ralph Gonzales of the University of Colorado Health Science Center in Denver.

- In the past 10 to 15 years, doctors have seen an epidemic of *streptococcus pneumonia* that is resistant to penicillin and penicillin derivatives, Gonzales said. The strain of bacteria is a leading cause of ear and sinus infection, meningitis and other common and potentially serious illnesses.

- Drug resistance has been blamed on overuse of antibiotics and the failure of some patients to take their medicine properly. Some patients stop taking their medication once they feel better but before the infection has been knocked out, enabling the hardiest germs to survive and multiply.

- In 1992, doctors prescribed antibiotics which are not effective to two-thirds of bronchitis sufferers who visited them in their offices and half of common-cold sufferers and patients with other upper respiratory infections, the researchers found.

- That amounted to 12 million prescriptions, or one in every five antibiotic prescriptions written for adults that year, the researchers said.

- The 1992 figures were the latest available for the study, but the 1995 numbers have since become available and are similar, Gonzales said.

- Doctors have been prescribing antibiotics for upper respiratory infections because until recently they thought that it wouldn't hurt, and that a very small chance existed that it might help, Gonzales said.

- In an accompanying editorial, Dr. Benjamin Schwartz of the Centers for Disease Control and Prevention said "an immediate and aggressive response" is needed to combat inappropriate prescribing of antibiotics.

- We encourage all physicians to examine their own practices and identify where they can decrease unnecessary antimicrobial use," he said.

- Patients can take the pressure off their doctors by putting up with the coughs that follow upper respiratory infections and can last for three weeks, Gonzales said.

- "Give your body's own immune system enough time to clear the infection," he said. Also, any patient who had been prescribed an antibiotic should consider asking the doctor: "Do you really think I need this?"

- In the study, rural doctors were about twice as likely as urban ones to prescribe an antibiotic for a cold, bronchitis or other upper respiratory infection, all other factors being equal.

- Gonzales speculated that because people in rural areas often travel a great distance to see doctors, the physicians may be trying to head off bacterial complications that could occur when the patients are back home.

- Also, he said, rural practices tend to be much busier because doctors are in short supply, so these physicians may feel too rushed to explain to patients why antibiotics are unnecessary.

Intestinal Flora

It's absolutely astounding to me that the Chicago [AP] report never mentioned the fact that the antibiotic prescribed by doctors just about destroys your intestinal flora. Just as medical schools have minimal courses on the benefits of nutritional supplements, they obviously overlooked the damages wreaked by antibiotics to your colon.

The bacteria found in the colon can be grouped into two categories based on their effect on humans. They're referred to as "friendly" or "unfriendly" bacteria. "Unfriendly" bacteria produce toxic by-products that contribute to long-term illness and chronic degeneration of the body. "Friendly" bacteria [also known as probiotics] favorably alter the intestinal flora balance, inhibit the growth of harmful bacteria, promote good digestion, boost immune function, and increase resistance to infection. People with flourishing intestinal colonies of beneficial bacteria are better equipped to fight the growth of disease-causing bacteria.

There are several trillion friendly bacteria comprising over 400 species in the average human gastrointestinal tract. While *lactobacillus acidophilus* is the most well known of these, others also play a crucial role in keeping us healthy. They include *lactobacillus salivarius/casei/rhamnosus, bifidobacterium bifidum/longum/lactis* and *streptococcus thermophilus*, among others. In a healthy colon the friendly bacteria outnumber the unfriendly, or pathogenic ones. Our colon can maintain its health with 15% unfriendly bacteria, if the body contains at least 85% probiotic friendly bacteria, such as the lactobacilli and *bifidobacteria* strains. Unfortunately, in most people this percentage is reversed.

What damages the flora balance?

Two of the most damaging substances to the delicate intestinal flora balance are chlorine and sodium fluoride, present in most treated city water, and thus in most commercial beverages including soft drinks. The consumption of coffee and alcoholic beverages further contributes to the destruction of the intestinal flora. **Antibiotics** [the opposite of probiotics], unhealthy eating habits and stress can also disrupt the natural ecology of the digestive tract. "In a study that was reported in the *Journal of Infection and Immunology*, it was found oral penicillin [*an antibiotic*] administered to experimental animals reduced the total population of anaerobic bacteria by a factor of 1,000 including beneficial bacteria which are called *lactobacilli* . . . . As the good bacteria are killed off, the potentially harmful bacteria increase rapidly. This study reported translocation of the harmful bacteria out of the intestinal tract and into the lymph nodes surrounding the intestinal tract. From these lymph nodes, these bacteria were then strategically placed to cause new infections throughout the body.

The intestinal microflora can be replenished with friendly bacteria by using probiotic supplements. These supplements are only effective if they're designed to withstand the extreme acidity of the stomach. Once the friendly bacteria reach the small and large intestines, they need dietary fiber to stay alive. A team of researchers from the Medical College of Georgia has been studying the link between fiber and bacteria. This is what one of the scientists, Dr. Ganapathy had to say: "You need to eat dietary fiber to provide the food for bacteria. Otherwise, they are not going to survive there. Antibiotics can wipe out good bacteria as well, leaving a void where disease-causing bacteria can grow."

"The gut is a huge immune organ; there are more immune cells in our gut than there are in the rest of the body put together," said Dr. Robert G. Martindale, a gastrointestinal surgeon with a special interest in probiotics.

Eating yogurt is not enough to ensure replenishment of beneficial bacteria.

If your doctor tells you to replace the destroyed intestinal flora his antibiotic prescription destroyed, run the other way,. He is far removed from the cutting edge.

Certain foods such as yogurt naturally contain *lactobacilli*, however, this may not be enough to keep the bad bacteria in check.

"Commercially available fermented foods are, unfortunately, unreliable as sources of *lactobacilli*," says Leo Galland, M.D., F.A.C.N., director of Foundation for Integrated Medicine, because the lactic acid and hydrogen peroxide which *lactobacilli* naturally produce may kill the producers themselves if their concentration becomes excessive. . . . The most reliable way to supplement your diet with *lactobacilli* is to buy nutritional supplements which have been tested by an independent outside laboratory and which list the concentration of viable bacteria found on culture. *Lactobacilli* are killed by heat, moisture and sunlight. The making of tablets generates heat which lowers the number of viable organisms. *Lactobacilli* should be freeze-dried, in powder or capsules, in opaque moisture-proof containers."

FOS – the food for beneficial bacteria

Friendly bacteria are living creatures which need nourishment to live and to multiply. When they receive nourishment, such as fiber, via the foods or supplements we take, they are able to maintain a stable population and can continue to play their crucial health-preserving role. Another favorite food of friendly bacteria is FOS [*fructooligosaccharides*]. Probiotic supplements that provide this food for the beneficial gut bacteria may, therefore, be more potent than just regular supplements.

Enteric coating

The stomach is a highly acidic environment that destroys all bacteria – the good ones as well as the bad. If the friendly bacteria from our supplements are abolished before they reach the intestines, where they are most needed, we will not enjoy their full benefits.

The way around this problem is to make the capsules containing the probiotics enteric-coated. This means that the capsules are coated with a special protective layer to ensure that the probiotic bacteria will survive through the stomach and make its way safely to the colon.

Selecting a premium quality probiotic supplement – Why Flora Protect Probiotics is highly recommended.

These are the hallmarks of a high-quality probiotic supplement:
• It contains several strains of viable bacteria that are either stable at room temperature, or refrigerated at all times [*Flora Protect* contains 8 different species of probiotics that are stable at room temperature; the stabilization system for the species was developed by the University of Wisconsin].

This ProBiotic is not enteric coated. I have been using Metagenics Ultra Flora Plus DF capsules for years and highly recommend the product. Each capsule has 15 billion organisms.

About those Crunches [not sit-ups]. They're easy to do [if done right]. It doesn't take long to do 100 reps. [work-up to that amount] and they may go a long way to rid you of that dangerous visceral fat you hear about which is not heart healthy.

Note: This chapter or any other chapter in this book is not meant to dispense medical advice or strategies for your health care. It is meant to raise your awareness to be pro-active to other health options which should be discussed with your health care professional.

CHAPTER 22

Find a Doctor Who can be an Interested Partner in Your Health Care

A close friend and my golf guru who is aware I am writing a book on alternative/ integrated/complementary health and knew I was writing a chapter on "Find a Doctor who can be an interested partner in your health care," gave me three articles from *Men's Health 2006*.

He said "you must read these before you write your chapter. It scared the hell out of me."
<u>Abstract from: "Survive Your Doctor," by T. E. Holt, M.D.</u>

- Average time a patient has to explain symptoms before doctor interrupts   18 seconds

- Percentage of doctors who have never had their patients' interview skills evaluated   80%

- Percentage of physicians who order unnecessary tests   79%

- Number of prescribing mistakes made annually that result in adverse reactions   51%

- Number of doctors who know another doctor they wouldn't trust with their lives   3 in 4

<u>Abstract from: "How to Get Out of the Hospital Alive," by Erin Hobda and Ted Spiker.</u>
<u>Identify the Best Hospital</u>

The time to decide where you want to be treated in a non-emergency situation is now – not when you're coping with a cancer diagnosis or wrestling with the reality of a blocked artery.

Start by visiting qualitycheck.org to see which hospitals in your area have been vetted by the national healthcare watchdog group, the Joint Commission on Accreditation of Health Care Organizations. Another good tactic: Go to MensHealth.com, keyword *doctor*, for a list of the 100 most-wired hospitals, which are probably using the latest information technology that helps reduce medical errors. If a particular hospital isn't on the list, call to see if it has one key advance: bar-coded processes for dispensing medications. Confirm that the correct drug is being given – a huge step in decreasing medication errors.

<u>When You're Admitted</u>

<u>Research your doctor</u>. Maybe you already know and trust the doctor handling your case. And if so, great. But if he's a stranger, run a basic background check to make sure he practices medicine, not mayhem. Go to docboard.org/docfinder.html, a site that provides links to every state's medical board or health department, and look for its database of physician profiles. In

addition to basic information on education, most of the sites also list disciplinary actions and malpractice claims.

Enlist a drug pro. You've probably never heard of a clinical pharmacist, but having one on your case can reduce the risk of medication errors and adverse drug reactions, according to a study review in the *Archives of Internal Medicine*. "They improve patient care by monitoring high-risk drugs, interacting directly with patients, and providing comprehensive medication instructions after discharge," says lead author Peter Kabeli, Ph.D. If the hospital doesn't employ a clinical pharmacist, ask if a staff pharmacist can perform some of the same functions.

Use a condom. A condom catheter, that is. University of Michigan researchers surveyed 75 men who had been catheterized using either an indwelling catheter or a condom catheter, which has a silicon sheath that fits over the penis. Not only were the condom catheters more comfortable, but the men who used them were half as likely as their counterparts to develop urinary-tract infections. They come in five sizes, so be picky about fit. Be sure to ask for a new one, not a sterilized one many hospitals use.

Flash your doctor. Grab your camera phone and take a photo of your physician. In a recent Mayo clinic study, researchers found that patients with a snapshot of their doctor were better able to identify him. This in turn may help cut down on the number of medical mistakes caused by giving information to the wrong medical personnel. [See, "Know Who's Who," below.]

Demand clean hands. A small percentage of healthcare workers are compulsively clean, but "others wash their hands only when they think they've gotten them dirty," says Gail Van Kanegan, R.N., C.N.P., coauthor of *How to Survive Your Hospital Stay*. Ask for a pump dispenser of alcohol-based hand sanitizer and put in on your night table – the staff will get the hint, as will your friends and family. Hand washing is a joint commission of accreditation for all hospitals.

While You're in a Hospital Bed

Know Who's Who. "Some patients assume that every man in a scrub suit is a doctor," says Dr. Pezzi, and they pass information to whoever comes in the room. But that guy could be a clueless medical technician, increasing the odds of a medical mistake. Make sure all people identify themselves, and convey changes in your condition only to doctors and nurses.

Check for leaks. If someone wears a surgical mask too loosely, air – and germs – can escape through the gaps. "Usually, it's the doctor doing it, not the nurses," says Dr. Pezzi. Look to see that their masks are snug.

Scope out the Stethoscope. While he's hearing your heartbeat, bacteria are hopping on your body. Ask your doctor to sanitize his stethoscope. Just as effective: a disposable glove over its diaphragm, or an antimicrobial coating called AgIon.

Sanitize yourself. The infection risks from sharing a toilet seat with an incontinent roommate are obvious. What isn't so apparent is the risk you pose to yourself. "More often, organisms that cause infections come from the patient's own homegrown flora," says Larson. Protect yourself by slathering your hands with that alcohol-based sanitizer as if your life depends on it.

Dose up on aspirin. Swallowing 325 milligrams a day can halve your risk of developing a staph infection, says Ambrose Cheung, M.D., a professor of microbiology at Dartmouth College. "Aspirin can activate the stress response of staph bacteria [including the superbug MRSA], which keeps it from adhering to your tissue." Ask your doctor and pharmacist before adding a medication to your drug regimen.

Protect your bed. Tell visitors that if they truly wish you a speedy recovery, they should take a seat in a chair, not on your sheets. In a study in the *British Medical Journal*, researchers found that a combination of infection-control strategies that included eliminating visitor contact with a patient's bed was able to stop the spread of MRSA and reduce the number of infections by 70 percent. "This is one measure that patients can really control,:" says Leela Biant, Ph.D., the lead author.

When the Nurse Comes Knocking

Pop the question. As in "How long have you been doing this?" The ideal nurse has been in the same unit, the same specialty, and the same hospital for more than a few years. [Don't assume that an older-looking nurse is the most experienced. "More people are going into nursing when they're 40 or 50, and they may be less experienced," says Sean Clarke, Ph.D., R.N., associate director of the University of Pennsylvania's Center for Health Outcomes and Policy Research.] Because of the current nursing shortage, you may not have much choice in terms of who cares for you, but if you have concerns about inexperienced nurses, talk to the nurse manager.

Rate response time. It's the most critical part of the nurse-patient relationship: They come when you call. If no one arrives within 2 or 3 minutes of when you pull the cord or push the button, your care could be compromised in an emergency. "You can't expect every request or concern to be acted on immediately, but every patient call needs to be checked out relatively quickly," says Clarke. As with the issue of experience, discuss slow response time with the nurse manager.

Be wary of bling. When scientists at Rush University Medical Center in Chicago analyzed the hands of 66 nurses, they found that the ring wearers had ten times more bacteria than the bare-fingered bunch. One theory is that bacteria colonize in the microscopic space between ring and skin, and are then protected from being washed away. Scan the hands of doctors, nurses, and anyone else who wants to touch your body, and request that any jewelry come off before a rescrub.

Triple-check your meds. Do it even if you're being shadowed by a clinical pharmacist. University of Pennsylvania researchers recently found that over the course of just 1 month, more than 25 percent of the 502 critical-care nurses evaluated had made at least one mistake, usually with medication. A nurse is supposed to double-check to make sure that the patient is receiving the correct medication; you can provide the triple-check by asking what it is and why you're getting it.

When Surgery is Scheduled

Run the numbers. If your surgeon seems too eager to operate, go to MensHealth.com, keyword *doctor*. There you can compare rates of the most commonly over-performed procedures by region, city, or hospital. "In some places, back-surgery rates are 10 times what they are in others. And it's not because the people there are 10 times more likely to have back problems," says Jon Skinner, Ph.D., a professor of family medicine and economics at Dartmouth College. "It means some doctors like to do back surgery and think it works, while others are more conservative." Or they're running a scam. A few years ago, the FBI arrested two cardiologists for doing hundreds of unnecessary bypasses.

Empty the O.R. Can too much care kill? A new Dartmouth study shows that the more money a hospital spends on a single patient's care, the poorer the outcome of the treatment. More cash means more physicians per patient, says Skinner, the lead author, "It's hard to get eight or nine doctors to agree and communicate well." Ask that unnecessary personnel such as medical residents be kept out of the O.R.

Get tucked in. Before you go under anesthesia, ask for an extra blanket. The combination of a cold operating room and anesthesia can lead to mild hypothermia, which can slow the posy-op healing process.

Confirm the cut. A few years ago, the Joint Commission on Accreditation of Healthcare Organizations created a new protocol to help reduce the chances of a surgical mistake. It's a smart system – assuming it's used , and used properly. Be sure that the mark indicating where to cut is . . .
- on the incision site. Writing "don't cut here" on a healthy area can look like "cut here" if the ink smudges.
- Direct – either a doctor's initials or "YES." An X is ambiguous – it could be read as "keep out" or "X marks the spot."
- Written in permanent marker that won't fade after your skin is washed and prepped for surgery.
- Written only by the surgeon.

Up the H_2O. Hydration equals healing. "In order for your body to heal, the cells must have sufficient amounts of water," says Van Kanegan, "If you're dehydrated, you're at risk of infection, pressure sores, electrolyte imbalances, heart irregularities, and other complications." Shoot for 8- to 12-ounce glasses of water a day in the weeks before your hospital visit. Water down the danger.

Abstract from: "The Junkie in the O.R.," by Christopher McDougall

With just one slip of the scalpel, a surgeon can accidentally cripple or end a person's life. But this isn't the most dangerous person in the operating room. Instead, it's the masked addict looking for a fix.

One of the most dangerous and best-kept secrets of the medical profession is the epidemic of anesthesiologists who are addicted to their own drugs. More than 400 drug-addicted anesthesiologists and residents may be working in operating rooms at this moment, based on the findings of separate studies by John Booth, M.D., a former Duke University anesthesiologist, and Mark S. Gold, M.D., a psychiatry professor at the University of Florida's McKnight Brain Institute.

That means, the next time you lie on an operating table and close your eyes, your odds of ever opening them again could be in the hands of someone who's injecting himself every 6 hours with fentanyl, a pain killer that's 100 times more potent than morphine. He'll be suspending you in a near-death state – slowing your heart, numbing your nerves, loosening your grip on consciousness – while simultaneously siphoning off drugs for himself and, at times, shooting up right in the middle of an operation. One mistake and you could end up dead, or in a never-ending coma.

Dr. Gold became aware of how many anesthesiologists were diverting drugs into their own veins while he was assessing 20 years' worth of confidential records at the Physicians Recovery Network, an intervention and rehabilitation organization. He was struck by how often "anesthesiology" turned up as an addicted doctor's specialty, so he began tabulating. Dr. Gold has been an addiction expert for more than 30 years, but even that didn't prepare him for the total: Anesthesiologists are overrepresented by a staggering 500 percent.

"We ran the numbers in a variety of permutations," Dr. Gold says, "and each way you look at it – year by year, consecutive cases, age group – it's clear that anesthesiologists are by far the most likely to have chemical-dependency problems."
Who's Hooked?

5 Signs of an Addicted Anesthesiologist

Before you go under, go online. At docboard.org/docfinder.html, you can check your state's medical board for malpractice cases and license actions. Very rarely will you meet your anesthesiologist before your procedure. So arrange to meet the anesthesiologist who is performing the procedure beforehand. After surveying more than 300 anesthesiology departments, British doctors developed a junkie profile. Watch for:

Cold or flu symptoms. Sure, the coughing and sweating could be legitimate symptoms – but then, why is he at work? Most doctors stay home when they have a touch of something.

Off-color comments. Narcotics relax your inhibitions. If your anesthesiologist sounds less like a doc and more like a shock jock, lean in for a closer look at those eyes.

Drug-addicted eyes. You aren't checking for a bloodshot gaze, but rather for pupil size. Pinpoint pupils could mean he's recently shot up, and dilated pupils often indicate withdrawal.

Mood swings. Because an addicted anesthesiologist needs a fresh shot every 3 hours or so, he can go from suave to snarly in the midst of explaining your procedure.

Excessive overtime. Try to find out from him [or a nurse] if he's the go-to guy when a volunteer is needed. Grabbing a lot of extra shifts may mean he's staying near his supply.

Medical Tests That Do More Than Improve Your Doctor's Fiscal Health

Don't be so free with your pee. Johns Hopkins University researchers recently found that during a typical doctor visit, 43 percent of patients will undergo at least one unnecessary test. Physicians do this to avoid malpractice suits or, more often, to pad their pockets, says Jon Skinner, Ph.D., a professor of family medicine and economics at Dartmouth College. Here's how we get probed for profit:

Urinalysis. The Johns Hopkins study showed that 37 percent of patients underwent an unwarranted urine test. "It might seem harmless, but a simple urine test can lead to an unnecessary biopsy, which can be painful, inconvenient, and potentially dangerous," says Dan Merenstein, M.D., the study's lead author.

MRIs. An abnormality will pop up in MRIs of the back in 84 percent of healthy people, Skinner says, which can lead to "a medical fishing expedition" involving further invasive testing and surgery.

Electrocardiograms. EKGs were the second most commonly overused test performed on healthy patients in the Johns Hopkins study, and previous research has shown that 20 percent result in false-positive diagnoses.

X-rays. An x-ray may not nuke you the way a CT scan can, but it's still radiation. Be on guard if the doctor's office has a machine.

Full-body CT scans. They aren't as accurate as advertised, many insurers refuse to cover the cost [they can run you as much as $1,000], and research has shown that the amount of radiation your body is exposed to may increase your cancer risk.

Such horror stories have become shockingly familiar in American medicine.

Finding a Doctor, etc., etc.

In my research I have read many interesting approaches to choosing a doctor. I am sure all of my readers have a doctor and/or doctors to meet their healthcare issues that they have been using for years and have basically a strong sense of confidence in him or her but feel on occasion something is lacking.

This is one of the interesting approaches to find out if your doctor's attitude is to become a partner in your healthcare or just has a condescending manner.

Dr. Ronald Hoffman, a well-regarded alternative /complementary health physician as well as author and radio personality offers an interested sacrosanct in his book on how to choose your doctor.

How open is your present doctor to integrative medicine?

• Excellent response

Doctor's Responses: "I encourage you to participate in your care by researching and applying alternative approaches to your condition – let's talk about what might be most helpful and compatible with your conventional treatment. If you prefer, we'll use standard medicine only as a last resort."
Grade: Excellent
Suggested Action: Congratulations! You've found an ideal "health coach" who will supervise and support your wellness efforts.

• Good response

Doctor's Responses: "I'm somewhat familiar with these approaches. I believe some work, some don't, and some could be downright harmful. I'll try to get information on how the alternatives you're taking could interact with my standard treatments – my goal is just to keep you safe."
Grade: Good
Suggested Action: Encourage your doctor to partner with you and provide detailed information on CAM treatments to bridge her/his knowledge gap.

• Fair response

Doctor's Responses: "I'm frankly skeptical about these 'alternatives' you're using, and admit I don't know much about them. I guess you can try them, but keep me informed, and I'll alert you to any possible interaction."
Grade: Marginal
Suggested Action: Inform your doctor that you would welcome a more accepting attitude. The situation is salvageable – but you will have to be tactful and proactive.

● Poor response

Doctor's Responses: "There you go about those *alternatives* again! When are you going to just accept that they're dangerous, unproven, and mostly rip-offs! If you keep on trying to play doctor, I'm afraid I won't be able to keep on treating you."
Grade: Unsatisfactory
Suggested Action: Vote with your feet!

<u>Source</u>: "How to talk with your Doctor." Dr. Ronald Hoffman.

Patients shouldn't tolerate what they see as high-handed or inconsiderate behavior on the part of a physician – long waits, rushed consultations, perfunctory examinations, brusque or evasive answers to questions. Nor should they tolerate a condescending or authoritarian attitude, or a doctor who blames them when treatments fail. Patients needn't endure office staff who are rude or inattentive or who consider it their job to shield the doctor from the patient.

Don't fire your physician in a moment of anger over an isolated incident, especially if the relationship has been a long and trusting one. Try discussing your grievances. Your doctor may not even know a problem exists. If the problem still can't be resolved, it's time to leave. Certain misdeeds, of course, shouldn't be forgiven even if they occur only once. Don't return to a doctor who misdiagnoses a significant problem or who fails to follow up an important abnormal laboratory result.

There's no sure way to find a new personal physician who will meet all your needs. But a few steps can help you avoid a poorly qualified physician – and just might lead you to the right person.

First you'll need some names. Many people simply ask a satisfied friend or relative. A better approach, in my view, is to ask a healthcare professional – a physician, nurse, therapist, technician, or social worker – who has seen many doctors in action. Almost anyone who works in a hospital can tell you which doctors are regarded highly by their patients and colleagues.

If you don't know an insider, call the local hospital and ask the medical staff secretary for the names of several family practitioners or internists on the roster who have agreed to take referrals for new patients. The county medical society can also provide names. Never rely on a paid advertisement in the newspaper or Yellow Pages.

Once you have a short list of candidates, investigate their qualifications. [If you have managed-care health insurance, see if your candidates are all "participating providers"]. Look into these areas:

<u>Resources for Funding an Integrated/Alternative Complementary Doctor</u>:

Consortium of Academic Health Centers for Integrative Medicine: www.imconsortium.org. Organization of academic medical centers offering integrative education, research, and care.

National Center for Complementary and Alternative Medicine:
www.nccam.hih.gov/health or [888] 644-6226. A division of the National Institutes of Health. Provides articles and databases of latest CAM research.

Second M.D. Opinion

A second opinion is even more important than in the past. Under pressure to hold down costs, some doctors may suggest a less expensive course of therapy when another approach might be more appropriate. Or they may be motivated to boost profits with a more costly alternative. In some cases, doctors base their advice not on scientific evidence but on their own clinical experience or that of their close colleagues. Or their advice may even reflect their confidence in their ability to perform a procedure successfully. A second opinion is one of the best ways for a patient to be sure that none of those biases will bar the way to the best possible treatment.

Unless it is an emergency situation, patients should seek a second opinion in the case of a recommended surgery or when a treatment strategy is not showing desired results in a reasonable time.

Even when there are no therapeutic alternatives to sort out, a second opinion can be of value. It can offer a fresh perspective if there's a vexing clinical problem. Or it can confirm a diagnosis or the wisdom of a course of treatment, and thus ease any doubts you – or your physician – may have.

When seeking another opinion, try not to go behind your physician's back, since the second physician will usually want to review data obtained during the original workup, thus avoiding unnecessary duplication. If you sense reluctance or defensiveness on your doctor's part, that's all the more reason to get a second opinion.

Remember, this is the only life you have and it's not a dress rehearsal. Have patience. Looking for the right doctor is analogous to crawling around in a haystack not knowing what a needle looks like.

Note: This chapter or any other chapter in this book is not meant to dispense medical advice or strategies for your health care. It is meant to raise your awareness to be pro-active to other health options which should be discussed with your health care professional.

CHAPTER 23

Paul's Tips for Everyday Living

A.   Top Anti-Inflammatory Super Foods

Beverages [Unsweetened]
Blueberry juice, cherry juice, green tea, pomegranate juice, vegetable juice

Fruit and Seeds [Raw, unsalted]
Almonds, flaxseeds, sesame seeds, walnuts

Fruit [Fresh and organic, if possible]
Apples, avocados, blueberries, cherries, grapefruit, oranges, pomegranates

Vegetables [Organic, if possible]
Arugula, asparagus, bell peppers, broccoli, cabbage, carrots, leeks, onions, romaine lettuce, scallions, shitake mushrooms, spinach, tomatoes

Herbs and spices
Basil, black pepper, cardamom, chives, cilantro, cinnamon, cloves, garlic, ginger, parsley, turmeric

Fish
Flounder, halibut [small], salmon [wild], scrod [available from *www.vitalchoice.com]*

Other
Egg whites, yogurt [plain, nonfat]

Source: Dr. Stephen Sinatra – *Heart, Health & Nutrition, May 2007*

A.   Aspirin

If you take low-dose aspirin for your heart, don't take ibuprofen [such as Motrin or Advil] often, since it can block the anti-clotting effect of the aspirin. According to a large new study of people with osteoarthritis, this interaction may increase the risk of heart attacks and strokes in those at high cardiovascular risk who are taking aspirin. Naproxen [such as Aleve] appeared to be safe. Last year the FDA warned about this ibuprofen/aspirin interaction. Occasional use of ibuprofen is okay, the FDA suggested, but you shouldn't take it during the 8 to 12 hours before or half hour after taking low-dose aspirin.

Source: University of California Berkeley Wellness Letter 10/07.

Alzheimer's Risk

Fatty Acid Found in Fish May Lower Dementia, Alzheimer's Risk

People with the highest blood levels of docosahexaenoic acid [DHA], an omega-3 fatty acid found in fish, may be less likely to develop dementia and Alzheimer's disease, according to a study in the November issue of the *Archives of Neurology*. Researchers studied 899 men and women [average age of 76] who had no dementia when the study began and followed them for an average of 9.1 years. The study participants were divided into quartiles based on their blood DHA levels. Compared to people in the lower three quartiles, those in the quartile with the highest DHA levels were 47 percent less likely to develop dementia and 39 percent less likely to develop Alzheimer's disease, the study found. And, among 488 participants who completed dietary questionnaires, those who reported eating fish more than twice a week were 39 percent less likely to develop dementia and 50 percent less likely to develop Alzheimer's disease than those who ate two servings or fewer weekly, the researchers reported.

Source: Men's Health Advisor, 2/07.

Test Your Antioxidant IQ

TRUE OR FALSE? To get the most antioxidants in your food, research findings say you should:

Always eat veggies raw. False. Tomatoes, carrots and spinach release more antioxidants when they are stir-fried, microwaved or lightly steamed. Add a little fat to increase antioxidant absorption.

Drink strong brewed hot tea, not iced tea. True. Ice dilutes the antioxidants, and storing tea in the fridge further depletes them. Instant and bottled teas offer few or no antioxidants.

Eat any kind of chocolate. False. White chocolate has no antioxidants; milk chocolate has few. Only dark chocolate has high levels.

Buy nuts with skins intact. True. Almond skins, for example, contain a lot of potent antioxidants.

Avoid frozen or canned food. False. Canned tomato sauces, paste and juice contain high amounts of lycopene, a potent antioxidant. Frozen [but not canned] fruits and vegetables generally match the antioxidant levels in their fresh counterparts.

Forget fruit juices-they are low in antioxidants. False. You can get high levels of diverse antioxidants in apple, grapefruit, cranberry and especially, purple grape juices.

Go for deep colors. True. Deep-green spinach and lettuces and the brightest berries provide the most antioxidants. Even black dried beans have more antioxidants than white or red beans.

Organic produce has more antioxidants. Don't count on it. The results of studies on this are unclear.

Source: Jean Carper – renowned health researcher.

B. **Blood Thinner Victim Featured on 20/20 Program**
By Robin Williams Adams – *The Ledger*

A local lawsuit by the family of a woman who died after receiving blood thinner 10 times greater than her doctor prescribed was featured on an ABC News 20/20 report.

Brian Ross and Rhonda Schwartz reported that a high-school student, working at a Walgreens in Lakeland, made a typing error that resulted in the higher doses.

Patient Beth Hippley had to stop taking chemotherapy for breast cancer when she had a massive stroke after taking the higher-dose medicine, ABC said in the 20/20 episode. It said she died earlier this year.

Legal actions are continuing in the 2003 case, according to records in the Polk County Clerk of the Court's office.

Pharmacists are expected to check prescriptions filled by pharmacy technicians, but the registered pharmacists failed to catch the error on Hippley's prescription, ABC said. Big chain stores hire thousands of pharmacy technicians, with some requiring only that students watch a short video before taking the job, ABC contends, raising concerns about the extent of pharmacy errors that aren't reported.

ABC said the local high school student testified that she watched a video and was taking classes in school to learn about the job.

Most states allow students to be employed if they are actively working for a GED or high school diploma, ABC said.

Lawyer Karen Terry, representing Hippley's family, said chains give "huge responsibility" to technicians who aren't adequately trained.

In a statement to ABCNews.com, Walgreens said, "We deeply regret the few errors that have occurred among the more than 500 million prescriptions we fill each year at our 5,600 pharmacies." Be sure you verify your doctor's prescriptions before you leave them at the pharmacy.

Robin Williams Adams can be reached at robin.adams@theledger.com or 863-802-7558.

Build Bones With Strength Training

Everyone knows strength training builds muscles, but did you know it also can help strengthen your bones? Researchers from the University of Arkansas analyzed a six-year, nationwide study that compared the effect of different activities on women's bone density. The results revealed that "weight-bearing activities" like strength training and yard work were linked to bone health, while activities such as swimming and jogging were found to have little effect on bone density.

"Weight-bearing exercises exert force on the bones," says lead researcher Lori Turner. "Like muscles, bone responds to force by growing. Muscles get larger, and bones become more dense."

People start to lose bone density between ages 30 and 40, so maintaining bone strength is beneficial for all. Of course, getting the recommended amount of calcium for your age is crucial. But also try picking up some dumbbells or spending a little time working in your garden to improve bone strength.

Source: FitSmart – Jorge Cruise.

Eating Bran Cereal, Then Popping a Multi

Bran binds to minerals such as zinc, magnesium and calcium, forcing them to be excreted instead of absorbed. And studies at New York City's St. Luke's-Roosevelt Hospital Center and elsewhere show that not getting enough of these essential nutrients can *double* the severity of PMS symptoms and the duration of colds, plus increase the risk of tension headaches, fatigue and even depression. "So rather than taking your multivitamin with breakfast, take it an hour before. Or, if that upsets your stomach, have it with lunch or dinner instead," suggests nutrition researcher Larrian Gillespie, M.D., author of *You're Not Crazy, It's Your Hormones* [Healthy Life Publications, 2003]. "But if you prefer taking vitamins with your first meal of the day, consider having your bran cereal as a bedtime snack."
Source: EatSmart-Jean Carper.

C.   Carpal Tunnel

Quick Cure for Carpal Tunnel Syndrome

If you suffer from carpal tunnel syndrome, Dr. Frank Shallenberg has great news for you. There's an easy way to treat it that really works wonders.

Carpal tunnel syndrome is an inflammation or swelling of the tendons of the wrist. Most people think that it's caused by repetitive motion. But that's only what triggers it. It's usually caused by a vitamin B2 [riboflavin] deficiency, a vitamin B6 [pyridoxine] deficiency, a cervical [neck] subluxation, excessive exposure to fluoride, and in rare cases, from the use of injectable growth hormone therapy.

The conventional treatment is to cease the offending activities, wear a wrist splint, or have a surgical decompression of the wrist tendons. Unfortunately none of these treatments addresses the real cause[s] of the disorder, and are often unsuccessful. Dr. Shallenberg found that employing treatments aimed at the causes is successful in over 90% of cases and it avoids the potential pitfalls of surgery. The best treatments consist of the following:

• Take a B-complex capsule containing 50 mg of each of the B-vitamins, along with 100 mg of vitamin B6, twice a day. You can expect to do this for three months before the problem resolves itself.

  • See an acupuncturist to reduce the wrist inflammation.

  • See a chiropractor to treat any cervical subluxation.

  • I like to inject a special form of B12 [methyl-B12] along with procaine and ozone just under the skin [sub-q] over the underside of the wrist once a week.

This works so well, most pain and irritation is gone in just a few weeks!

Source: Dr. Frank Shallenberger – Newsletter "Prescriptions for Healthy Living" 1/08.

I decided I would like verification from my own chiropractor of 12 years – *I have been going to chiropractors for over 33 years but I consider Dr. Steve Pruden [with offices in Manhattan and Roslyn, NY] the Zen master of chiropractors.* He totally agreed with the article.

D.   Drugs [Prescription]

When your doctor is prescribing a drug you never used before, have him split the quantity on two separate prescriptions.

Here is why:

1. Suppose he gives you a quantity for 3 months.
2. You become allergic after taking it for a short period of time.
3. Or it is not effective .

You have paid all of that money on a prescription drug that was of no benefit to you and you can't return.   *Source:* Paul's personal experience.

E.   Eyesight

Older adults with high levels of beta-carotene, vitamins C,D, and E, lutein, zeaxanthin, zinc, and omega-3, had healthier eyesight than those who had low levels of these nutrients, according to a new review of five large studies covering 21,485 participants, aged 50 to 80, in over a dozen research centers around the world, from 1988 through 2005.

In the U.S. National Eye Institute Age-Related Eye Disease Study [AREDS], participants with moderate to high risk of losing eyesight-a condition known as age-related macular degeneration, or AMD-who took a **daily combination of 15 mg of beta-carotene, 500 mg of vitamin C, 400IU of vitamin E, plus 80 mg of zinc oxide with 2 mg of copper [cupric] oxide, had an average 22% lower risk of developing AMD** than those who did not take these nutrients. The placebo group had the highest risk of AMD. Doctors included the 2 mg of copper to protect against copper deficiency, which can occur when zinc levels are high.

Participants in the Netherlands based Rotterdam Study, who had high levels of beta-carotene, vitamins C and E, and zinc, had substantially lower risk for AMD than those with low levels.

In the 20th report of AREDS **participants who had high levels of the omega-3 docosahexaenoic acid [DHA] were less likely to develop** the most serious type of **AMD**, called "wet" AMD, where abnormal blood vessels form in the eye.

In two studies, the Carotenoids in Age-Related Eye Disease Study [CAREDS] and the Pathologies Oculaires Liees a l'Age [POLA] **in participants with AMD, the disease progressed more slowly for those who had a high level of lutein or zeaxanthin** compared to those with low levels.

In the National Health and Nutrition Examination Survey [NHANES], **those with the highest levels of vitamin D had 40% less risk of developing AMD** than those who had the lowest levels.

Source: Current Opinion in Ophthalmology: 2007; Vol.18,220-3.

F.   5 Fat Fighters That Really Work

Some fat-busting supplements do work, Harry Preuss, MD, reports in a new book, *The Natural Fat-Loss Pharmacy.* The Georgetown University Medical Center researcher says the following may help you lose and keep off weight and fat [you still need to restrict calories]:

- **EGCG**, an antioxidant in green tea, increases metabolism to burn calories, kills fat cells and blocks formation of new ones. What to take: a green tea extract pill before meals for a total daily dose of 270 mg to 325 mg of EGCG.
- **CLA**, conjugated linoleic acid, can melt body fat and build muscle without calorie counting or exercise. What to take: 1.7 g, twice a day of Tonalin CLA.
- **HCA,** Hydroxycitric acid, derived from a tropical fruit, quadrupled weight loss in an eight-week moderate diet. What to take: 1,500 mg, three times a day, 30 minutes before meals. The brand Preuss tested, Super CitriMax, is available from Now Foods.
- **Chromium** targets the loss of fat instead of muscle. What to take: For weight loss, 200 mcg, three times a day, of chromium bound to niacin [ChromeMate], or chromium picolinate or histidinate. For maintenance, take 200 mcg a day.
- **Starch Blockers** cut absorption of carbs. What to take: CarbEase or brands with the ingredient Phase 2. Follow label directions.

Source: Jean Carper, renowned authority on nutrition.

F.   Fruits and Vegetable Serving

What is a Serving?

Fruits

- 1 medium apple, banana or orange
- ½ cup of chopped or canned fruit
- ¾ cup of whole fruit juice

Vegetables

- 1 cup of raw leafy vegetable
- ½ cup of other vegetables, cooked or chopped raw
- ¾ cup of vegetable juice

How Many Servings Do You Need a Day?

Calories/day	Fruit	Vegetable	Total
2,800 [active men]	4	5	9
2,200 [sedentary men]	3	4	7
1,800 [inactive older men]	2	3	5

Source: Men's Health Advisor 3/02.

G. Grapefruit Juice and Prescription Drugs: Some Dangerous Interactions

The January 5th issue of the *Medical Letter,* a widely respected source of independent information about pharmaceuticals and dietary supplements, has a review of the increasingly researched problem of the interaction between grapefruit juice and many prescription and over-the-counter drugs. Like most interactions between chemicals in the body, this one involves the impairment, by grapefruit juice, of the body's [intestines] ability to metabolize many drugs, leading to higher than expected-and sometimes dangerous-levels of these drugs. According to the *Medical Letter,* the enzyme inhibited by grapefruit juice, leading to the impairment of metabolizing drugs, "is involved in the metabolism of about half of all drugs currently prescribed."

Addressing the issue of whether you can avoid this problem by drinking grapefruit juice at a time other than when you take your medicines, the article went on to say that, "because grapefruit juice is at least partly an irreversible inhibitor, . . . the activity of the enzyme does not immediately return to normal after the juice has moved through the intestine. Interactions with drugs, therefore, cannot be fully avoided by taking them at a different time. The recovery half-life. . . after a single glass of grapefruit juice appears to be about one day, and after three days little inhibitory effect remains. . . One glass a day for three days doubled serum concentrations of lovastatin [the cholesterol-lowering drug, MEVACOR]."

H. Hemorrhoids

Most people during their lifetime have experienced hemorrhoids. This recommendation is for people who have chronic hemorrhoid problems.

Hemorrhoids, as you know, occur in the rectum/anus area. This area contains a network of blood vessels known as the internal and external rectal plexus.

These blood vessels become enlarged when subjected to either constant or intermittent pressure caused by a variety of factors, including: straining during bowel movements, overweight, pregnancy, or strenuous physical activity. Chronic constipation, brought on by a low-fiber diet, can also lead to hemorrhoid disease.

Often, hemorrhoids left untreated progress to the point where the only solution is surgery.

Approximately 123,000 Americans must undergo hemorrhoid surgery a year. Millions more self-medicate, often with little or no relief using nonprescription ointments and suppositories.

Source: Abstracted and edited, Hemorrhoid Relief Center www.hemmorrhoidcenters.com

Grape seeds *in the form of OPCs* may be the answer for you.

Warning: *If you eat a diet laced with refined carbohydrates, very low fiber and read "Gone with the Wind" while you're on the john, this may not help.*

My chiropractor Steve Pruden recommended grape seed extract to me 4 years ago. I have never used *Preparation H* again. At that time I was not familiar with OPCs, which happen to be more expensive than grape seed extract. But the formula is advertised to be far more effective.

Grape Seed Extract 101
"There is no relevant pharmaceutical nutritional, biochemical or analytical definition of a 'grape seed extract,' nor is there one standardized manufacturing method."

Author: After researching that information, I felt OPCs were the best form to take.
Quoted from FLAVAY, manufacturers of a supplement containing OPCs. Patented by Dr. Masquelier in France.

Dr. Masquelier has patented a process to isolate the formula for proanthocyanidin (OPCs) from grape seeds.

The factors contained in grape seeds extract provide a broad spectrum of antioxidant protection.

It does not end there.

Scientific studies document multiple effects, including antibiotic, anti-tumor, anti-diabetic, anti-ulcer, pro-heart and arteries, and anti-brain aging.

Source: abstracted and edited from *Life Extension* 7/05; www.herbal-powers.com/ grapeseed.html. abstracted.

Studies suggest that the active components of grape seeds [*author: bear in mind is that grape seed extract is a much more potent form of grape seeds and therefore more effective. OPCs are much more potent.*] inhibit the destruction of collagen structures. Healthy collagen are very important to the overall health of any capillaries. [*Author: This is where the grape seed was effective in curing my hemorrhoid problem.*]

Conclusion

Four years ago I took 300 mg of grape seed extract with great results in approximately 4-6 weeks.

Since researching OPCs [*I switched from grape seed extract*], I use **Nature's Way**. They use Dr. Masquelier's patented formula [*you take the tablets based on your body weight*]. The cost is $22.39 for 90 tabs. If you use the FLAVAY brand, the cost is $48.75 for 60 tabs.

H.   Hot Flashes
Author: *Health News Letter*
Posted: 1/11/2008

- **Soybean compound may reduce hot flashes**

Boston, Jan. 10. A compound in soybeans might help reduce hot flashes in menopausal women, a U.S. study found.

The study, published in *Menopause*, found women taking a soy supplement reduced the frequency of hot flashes by more than 50 percent compared to a 39 percent reduction in the placebo group.

"What we are trying to find is a safe and effective alternative to hormone therapy," said author Dr. George Blackburn of Beth Israel Deaconess Medical Center and Harvard Medical School aid in a statement, "Our study found that patients who consumed the soy supplement showed a reduction in the number of hot flashes."

The researchers divided 147 menopausal women into three groups to compare the placebo to two concentrations of the compound in soybeans – daidzein-rich isoflavone-aglycone. After 12 weeks, hot flash frequency was reduced by 52 percent in the 40 mg DRI group and 51 percent in the 60 mg DRI group.

Isoflavones are one of several classes of phytoestrogens – substances with chemical structure similar to estrogen that exert both estrogen-like and anti-estrogen properties.

The study used a standardized, concentrated isoflavone ingredient called AglyMax made by extracting the isoflavones from soy germ fermented with Koji fungus.

Ads by Google for hot flashes:
Relief from Hot Flashes
Estrogen® can help reduce symptoms of menopause including hot flashes.
www.estroven.com

Menopausal Hot Flashes?
Our Personal Program has helped thousands of women, naturally.

www.womentowomen.com

"I Cured My Menopause"
Simple 5 Step Plan Using Groceries From Local Store – Works in Days
www.MenopauseDefeated.com

I.   Immune System

Six Immune Boosting Supplements

Garlic	2 cloves garlic [preferred], or 600-900 mg high-allicin content garlic.	Kyolic Great Earth's Odorless Garlic
Omega-3 fatty acids	500 mg fish oil [200 mg EPA/300 mg DHA]	Advanced Bio Solutions Norwegian Fish Oil
Quercetin	Eat apples and onions; drink tea, especially black tea; and/or take 300-500 mg in supplement form	TwinLab Allergy Fifhters Great Earth Bioflavanoid Complex Advanced BioSolutions Seasonal Solutions
N-acetylcysteine	600 mg or 1,200 mg in divided doses when ill. Most effective when taken on an empty stomach.	TwinLab NAC Life Extension N-Acetyl Cysteine
Coenzyme Q10	30-60 mg in softgel form or 100-200 mg in capsule form	Advanced BioSolutions Q-Gel Swanson Ultra CoQ10 Country Life Maxi Sorb C0Q10
L-carnitine	250-500 mg	Advanced BioSolutions Q-Gel Plus Solar L-carnitine

Recommended dosage [all on a daily basis unless otherwise noted.]
Source: Dr. Stephen Sinatra, *Heart, Health & Nutrition*, 12/01.

L.   Liver Failure

Safe Pain Reliever Causes 40% of Acute Liver Failure!

Acetaminophen is the active ingredient in painkillers [such as Tylenol], cough medicines, sleep aids, and more than 400 over-the-counter [OTC] and prescription products. When used correctly, it is one of the safest and most effective drugs on the market.

So why did a recent major study find that acetaminophen accounted for nearly 40% of patients hospitalized for acute liver failure? That's far more than any other cause of liver failure, and a great concern because liver damage can happen very quickly and may prove fatal without a liver transplant.

The Fine Line Between Safe and Deadly

Overdosing on acetaminophen is easier than with other painkillers. The recommended daily maximum dosage is 4,000 mg [4g] daily. Exceeding this by only 20% for even one day can result in liver injury and rapidly deteriorating liver function in healthy people. Some recover completely with proper treatment, while others will die without a liver transplant.

Avoid These 4 Common Mistakes

1. **Inadvertently taking two products** with acetaminophen together. Since the drug is found in over 400 products, you can easily exceed the maximum dosage.

2. **Thinking "more is better."** Many people deliberately take more than the recommended dosage or take the next dose too soon after the previous one.

3. **Combining alcohol with acetaminophen.** Alcohol increases production of the enzyme that makes acetaminophen toxic to the liver. If you drink alcohol and take acetaminophen you can overdose even at the recommended dosage.

4. **Taking it for much longer** than the recommended period of time. If you are in chronic pain, talk to your doctor. There are often much safer and more effective alternatives.
    Source: Health After 50 – A Johns' Hopkins Health Letter.

N.   Non-Steroidal Anti-Inflammation Drugs [NSAIDs]

According to the June 1999 issue of the *New England Journal of Medicine*, anti-inflammatory drugs account for more than 16,000 deaths a year due to intestinal hemorrhaging. "If deaths from gastrointestinal toxic effects from NSAIDs [nonsteroidal anti-inflammation drugs] were tabulated separately in the National Vital Statistics reports, these effects would constitute the fifteenth most common cause of death in the United States. Yet these toxic effects remain mainly a silent epidemic, with many physicians and most patients unaware of the magnitude of the problem. Furthermore, the mortality statistics do not include deaths ascribed to the use of over-the-counter NSAIDs.
Source: Ultra Prevention, written by Mark Hyman and Mark Liponis, M.D.s.

Other information about Non-Steroidal Anti-Inflammatory Drugs [NSAIDs]

Aspirin is an NSAID medicine but it does not increase the chance of a heart attack Aspirin can cause bleeding in the brain, stomach, and intestines. Aspirin can also cause ulcers in the stomach and intestines. Some of these NSAID medicines are sold in lower doses without a prescription [over-the-counter]. Talk to your healthcare provider before using over-the-counter NSAIDs for more than 10 days.

Source: Pfizer Pharmaceuticals.

O.   You Can Prevent Osteoporosis
Taking vitamin D along with calcium keeps bones strong.

If I were to ask what's the best way of keeping your bones healthy, what would you say? You've probably heard about the role that calcium plays, but did you know that vitamin D is just as crucial?

People who lose bone mass at an accelerated rate eventually may develop osteoporosis, a medical condition characterized by weak bones that break easily. Folks with this condition suffer not only from the pain of fractures but also from deformities that accompany a weakened skeletal frame. We've all seen elderly men and women who are stooped over so much that they can't straighten up. This represents the disease in its worst form. And really, the time to address osteoporosis is long before it gets to that stage.

Although aging is a risk factor for developing osteoporosis, it's not inevitable that we will end up with brittle bones. Let's explore two simple but effective supplement strategies that can put the odds in our favor.

CALCIUM. Any program to prevent osteoporosis must include adequate amounts of calcium because it's a basic component of bone. We may think of bones as stable structures, but in fact they are quite active. The two primary types of bone cells, osteoblasts and osteoclasts, work in opposition to one another. Osteoblasts build new bone, while osteoclasts tear it down through resorption. When we're under age 30 or so, bone-building osteoblastic activity rules, so bones get stronger. But as we get older, the balance of activity in our bones shifts toward the resorbing osteoclasts, making bones thinner and weaker. For some people this shift is accelerated, and the long, slow road to osteoporosis begins.

A diet that doesn't have adequate amounts of calcium contributes to the bone thinning. Recommendations have changed over time, but here's a good rule of thumb for adults: 1,000 mg a day for those under 50 and 1,200 mg a day for those over 50. Of course, this is for prevention, not treatment, of osteoporosis. People who already show evidence of thinning bones will require more.

P.   Protecting the Prostate and "Going" problems

Men who had high levels of selenium, multivitamins, vitamin E, and soy isoflavones had lower risk for prostate cancer than men with low levels of these nutrients in two new studies, and **soy isoflavones slowed the growth of prostate cancer cells** in a third new study.

In the selenium study, researchers measured the blood fluid [serum] levels of selenium in 724 men with prostate cancer and in 879 healthy men of the same age who entered the study at the same time, and followed up for eight years. Scientists found that **men who had higher selenium levels who also reported taking multivitamins had 39% lower risk for prostate cancer** than men with the lowest selenium levels. Doctors also found that **men with higher**

selenium levels who reported taking more than 28 IU of vitamin E per day had 42% lower risk for prostate cancer than men with the lowest selenium levels. Men with higher selenium levels who did not take vitamin E or multivitamins did not have significantly lower prostate cancer risk than those with low selenium levels.

In the soy isoflavone study, published March, 2007, the *Cancer Epidemiology Bio-markers & Prevention*, researchers examined the diets of 43,509 Japanese men, aged 45 to 74, average age 57, and followed up for nine years. During the study period, 307 men developed prostate cancer. Doctors found that **men who took 32.8 mg or more of soy isoflavones per day had 40% lower risk for prostate cancer** compared to men who took less than 13.2 mg per day. When doctors analyzed **men aged 60 or older**, leaving out the younger men, those **who took 32.8 mg or more of soy isoflavones per day had 49% lower risk for prostate cancer** compared to men who took the least soy isoflavones.

Source: *American Journal of Clinical Nutrition*: 2007, vol. 85, no. 1, 2009-17.

If you have a "going problem"

One of the pharmaceutical industry suggestions is, you take Avodart. One of the manufacturers cautions it may take 3 to 6 months for the medicine to work.

Some of the possible side effects are impotence, decreased interest in sex, breast tenderness or enlargement. Symptoms of an allergic reaction include rash, itching, swelling, dizziness or trouble breathing.

Instead of using Avodart I researched nutritional supplements [*that was after I was assured by my doctor there were no other prostate issues*].

I came up with this formula and it works for me, provided I don't drink large quantities of liquids past 8 P.M. I am good till 6:30 to 7:30 A.M.

(1) Saw Palmetto extract   375 mg
(1) Lycopene   15 mg
(1) Stinging Nettle   275 mg
(1) Pygem   10 mg
(1) Zinc   25 Mg

S.   Sugar Boosts Cancer Risk

Eating too much sugar can boost your risk of pancreatic cancer, one of the most deadly cancers, say Swedish researchers. They found that men and women who ate the most sugar [added to foods such as coffee, tea and cereal] were 69% more likely to develop pancreatic cancer than those who ate the least amount of sugar. Even worse: drinking more than two soft drinks a day, the main source of sugar for Americans, nearly doubled the odds of getting pancreatic cancer.

Researchers explain that sugar is rapidly absorbed into the bloodstream, driving up glucose and insulin levels. Excess glucose can actually poison and kill pancreatic cells, increasing cancer risk. Too much insulin results in insulin-like growth factor, which is thought to promote cell proliferation and cancer.

Source: Jean Carper, renowned nutritional researcher.

T.   To Your Health: Places to get more information on Aging and Health

- AARP, aarp.org/health/fitness
- American College of Sports Medicine [317] 637-9200
- Medline Plus, medlineplus.gov
- National Institute on Aging Information Center [800] 222-2225
- National Institute of Health [800] 311-3435
- Senior Health Care, myseniorhealthcare.com
- WebMD, webmd.com
- Yoga, ABC-of-yoga.com

Fit over 50	
Here is a recipe for fitness after 50 from AARP. It advises that any good fitness regimen should be geared toward:	*And it also suggests activities for these goals.*
• *Endurance.* To boost heart rate for an extended period of time	• Hiking, stair climbing, swimming, dancing, cycling, brisk walking, martial arts, volleyball, basketball, tennis
• *Strength.* To build muscle and make bones stronger	• Calisthenics or weight machines that work upper and lower body, martial arts, Pilates, rowing, cycling, hiking
• **Flexibility.** Stretching and increasing your range of motion	• Yoga, ballet, Pilates, martial arts, calisthenics
• *Balance.* To maintain posture and keep you from falling	• Yoga, tai chi, weight machines, posture exercises

V.   Vitamins "Yeses" and "Nos" You Should Know
      [Abstracted from *Earl Mendel's Vitamin Bible*]

[This is only a partial list and should be reviewed with your health professional.]

1. Vitamin A
    - A deficiency of Vitamin A can lead to loss of Vitamin C.
    - Large doses of Vitamin A may cause birth defects, particularly if taken in the first trimester, and should be avoided by pregnant women.
    - Don't engage in strenuous physical activity within four hours after taking Vitamin A if you want optimum absorption.
    - Vitamin A should not be taken in conjunction with the acre drug Acutane [isotretinoin].
    - Broad spectrums of antibiotics should not be taken with high doses of Vitamin A.

2. B Vitamins
    - An overingestion of Vitamin B-1 [thiamine] can affect thyroid and insulin production or might cause V-6 deficiency as well as loss of B vitamins.
    - Prolonged ingestion of any B vitamins [that are not full range] can result in significant depletion of others.
    - Pregnant women should check with their doctors before taking sustained doses of over 50 mg of Vitamin B6 [predoxine].
    - B-6 should not be taken by anyone under L-dopa treatment for Parkinson's disease.
    - B-2 [riboflavin]. Large doses should not be taken without antioxidants supplements, as it may cause a sensitivity to sunlight.
    - Biotin. Eating raw eggs deactivates the body's biotin.

3. C-Vitamins
    - Diabetes and heart patients should check with their doctors because Vitamin C might necessitate a lower dosage of pills.
    - Megadoses of Vitamin C wash out B-12 and folic acid, so be sure you are taking at least the daily requirements for both.
    - Excessive doses of choline, taken over a long period of time, may produce a deficiency of Vitamin B-6.
    - Inform your doctor if you are taking large amounts of Vitamin C. Vitamin C can change results of lab tests for sugar in the blood and urine and give false negative results for blood in stool specimens.
    - Diets might in fact increase phosphorous absorption and lower your calcium levels.
    - Calcium can interfere with the effectiveness of tetracycline.

4. D-Vitamins
    - If you have any heart issues, review with your health care professional the right dosage for you.
    - Milk that contains synthetic Vitamin D can deplete the body of magnesium.

- High doses of Vitamin D or calcium ascorbate are contraindicated if you are on the heart medication digoxin [lanoxin].

5. Vitamin E
   - Anyone with overactive thyroid, diabetes, high blood pressure, or rheumatic heart disease should consult with their health care professional before taking it.
   - If you take an iron supplement [ferroces sulfate], you are losing Vitamin E.

6. Folic Acid
   - High doses of folic acid for extended periods of time are not recommended for anyone with convulsive disorders or hormone-related cancer.
   - Folic acid and PABA might inhibit the effectiveness of sulforamides, such as gantrisis.
   - Folacin [folic acid] decreases the anticonvulsant actions of phenitoin [dilantin].

7. Miscellaneous
   (a) High doses of manganese can cause motor difficulties and weakness in certain individuals.
   (b) Too much sodium can cause a potassium loss.
   (c) Excessive zinc intake can result in iron and copper losses.
   (d) If you ad zinc to your diet, make sure you're getting enough Vitamin A.
   (e) Oyster shells, dolomite and bone meal, although sources of calcium, may contain lead or other toxic substances.
   (f) Antibiotics are reduced in their effectiveness when taken with supplements. [Take supplements at least an hour before or two hours after prescription antibiotics.

Note: This chapter or any other chapter in this book is not meant to dispense medical advice or strategies for your health care. It is meant to raise your awareness to be pro-active to other health options which should be discussed with your health care professional.

APPENDIX

Major Medical Accomplishments

- 1796. First vaccination against smallpox by Edward Jenner.
- 1730. First tracheotomy for treatment of diphtheria performed by George Martine.
- 1810. Samuel Hahnemann introduces homeopathy.
- 1819. French Doctor René Lavennec invented the first prototype stethoscope, a rolled-up tube of cylindrical paper.
- 1841. Ether was used as an anesthetic.
- 1847. Formation of the American Medical Association [AMA].
- 1852. George Cammann perfected the design of the stethoscope which then became the standard for commercial production.
- 1860. Louis Pasteur invented the microscope.
- 1895. Wilhelm Roentgen invented the ex-ray machine.
- 1897. Bayer perfected the aspirin.
- 1899. Defibrillation invented by Prevost and Batelli at the University of Geneva, Switzerland.
  - 1960. Professor Frank Partridge of Belfast, Ireland introduced portable defibrillators in ambulances.
  - 2003. Defibrillators were required by law in all Schools in New York State by law § 10577 signed by then Governor Pataki.
    Why were children's lives in harm's way from heart attacks for 43 years before this law was passed? That's anybody's guess!
- 1903. Madame Currie discovered radium, opening a new area of medical knowledge relative to the treatment of diseases.
- 1927. Philip Drinker & Louis Shaw developed the "iron lung."
- 1928. A Scottish medical researcher, Alexander Fleming, discovered penicillin.
- 1929. EEG Electronic encephalograph was perfected.
- 1937. Yellow fever vaccine developed by Max Theiler.
- 1940. Penicillin was perfected by Howard Forey.
- 1943. Kidney dialysis machine was built by Dutch physician Wilhelm Kloff.
- 1948. Cortisone. Merck Pharmaceutical synthesized compound E now known as cortisone.
- 1952. John Gibbons successfully developed Heart-Lung machine.
- 1953. Douglas Bevis developed implantation of artificial heart valve in open heart surgery.
- 1954. First successful kidney transplant.
- 1955. Open heart surgery. The two main pioneers were Walter Lelleha and Doctor John Kirklin.
- 1956. Cardio Pulmonary Resuscitation [CPR].
- 1957. Coenzyme C 10 discovered by Dr. Frederick Crane, a plant physiologist at the University of Wisconsin Enzyme Institute.

- 1958. Coenzyme Q 10. Doctor D. E. Wolf, assisting Doctor Karl Folkers at Merck Laboratories, first described the chemical structure of CQ 10, received the Priestly medal from the American Society for his research.
- 1958. Pacemaker,
- 1960. Oral contraceptive.
- 1963. Prevention of strokes.
- 1967. First heart transplant by Doctor Christian Barnard.
- 1970. First vaccine for Rubella.
- 1976. F.D.A.'s Cosmetics Act approved the use of leeches. The use of leeches in medicine goes back to Ancient Egypt 2500 years ago. Today, medical leeches are used in conjunction with microsurgery.
- 1981. AIDS first recognized.
- 1983. First successful human embryo transfer.
- 1986. Human genome project set up.
- 2003. Carolo Urbani of Doctors Without Borders alerted the World Health Organization to the threat of the SARS virus, triggering the most effective response to an epidemic in history. Urbani succumbs to the disease himself in less than 9 months after making the alert.

Source: Amalgamation of Abstracts from: w/Kipedia, Cambridge History of Medicine, Western Medicine, Medical Milestones of the Last Millennium.

INDEX

A

B

INDEX (continued)

INDEX (continued)

INDEX (continued)

INDEX (continued)

INDEX (continued)

About the Author

The motivation for writing this book was generated from Paul Boucher's disillusionment and frustration with traditional medicine's failure in properly treating his mother's illnesses which contributed to her premature death at 51.

This motivation became further galvanized due to the sub-par traditional medical care given to him by his good friend and internist of 20 years, which he strongly believes has left him with aortic valve and carotid artery stenosis.

He researched the three largest booksellers in the country – Borders, Barnes & Noble and Amazon.com. There were not any books that addressed the nine silent assailants in one single book, nor had they used his ground level language to explain these risk factors.

After Paul's discharge from the U.S. Marine Corps, he has been in the construction and real estate industry for over 50 years. He was accepted by the New York Department of Education [to qualify under the equivalent experience provisions, in lieu of a 5-year Master's Degree in Architecture] to sit for the New York State Registered Architect Exam and was Architectural Chair for five years for the Architectural Review Board in Manorhaven, New York. He has his Bachelor of Arts degree from Adelphi University in Garden City, New York.

Paul is very proud of his 17-year affiliation with the National Ski Patrol as a volunteer ski patrolman and his national appointment. He has patrolled at Windham Mountain, New York, and Magic Mountain, Bromley Mountain and Stratton Mountain, all in Vermont. He is currently working as a volunteer arbitrator for attorney-clients fee disputes in the New York Supreme Court system and has participated in mediating in small claims court as well as arbitrating in New York State lemon law cases for the New York State Attorney General's Office.

www.ingramcontent.com/pod-product-compliance
Lightning Source LLC
Chambersburg PA
CBHW081112170526
45165CB00008B/2428